ENHANCING SUCCESS OF ASSISTED REPRODUCTION

Edited by **Atef M.M. Darwish**

Enhancing Success of Assisted Reproduction
http://dx.doi.org/10.5772/3308
Edited by Atef M.M. Darwish

Contributors

Jozsef Daru, Attila Kereszturi, Atef Darwish, Micah J. Hill, Anthony M. Propst, Andrey Momot, Inna Lydina, Lyudmila Tsyvkina, Oksana Borisova, Galina Serdyuk, Murid Javed, Essam Michael, Michael Kamrava, Mei Yin, Mohamad E. Ghanem, Laila A. Al-Boghdady

Published by InTech
Janeza Trdine 9, 51000 Rijeka, Croatia

Publishing Process Manager Sandra Bakic
Technical Editor InTech DTP team
Cover InTech Design team

Additional hard copies can be obtained from orders@intechopen.com

Enhancing Success of Assisted Reproduction, Edited by Atef M.M. Darwish
p. cm.
ISBN 978-953-51-0869-6

For EU product safety concerns:
IN TECH d.o.o., Prolaz Marije Krucifikse Kozulić 3, 51000 Rijeka, Croatia,
info@intechopen.com or visit our website at intechopen.com.

Meet the editor

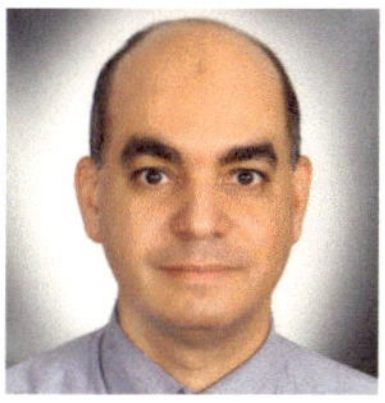

Dr. Atef M.M. Darwish graduated from Assiut School of Medicine in 1985 with an excellent grade and first class honors. He completed a residency in Obstetrics and Gynecology at the departments of Obstetrics and Gynecology, Assiut and Ain-Shams universities in 1986-1989. He got his Master degree in 1989 with Excellent degree. Between 1992-1994, he spent 2 years at the Endoscopic Unit of Ulm University, Germany. Thereafter, he received his Medical Doctorate in 1995 through a combined program between the University of Ulm, Germany and the University of Assiut, Egypt with Excellent degree. In 2009, he got a PhD degree in the reproductive medicine at the University of Utrichet, The Netherlands. Currently, he is Professor of Obstetrics and Gynecology, Faculty of Medicine, Assiut University. Moreover, he is a consultant of Obstetrics and Gynecology in three hospitals and he is the moderator and lecturer of many endoscopic societies. He authored an internationally registered undergraduate book (Practical Obstetrics and Gynecology) and edited two InTech multi-author books. He presented more than 70 presentations in national and international meetings, and published more than 45 papers in international medical journals, and 7 papers in national journals. His special interest has been in the area of gynecologic laparoscopy and hysteroscopy, reproductive medicine, and assisted reproduction. He published some innovative procedures in the field of endoscopic surgery and drug therapy of hyperprolactinemia.

Contents

Preface IX

Chapter 1 **The Role of Endoscopy in Management of Infertility 1**
Jozsef Daru and Attila Kereszturi

Chapter 2 **Endoscopy versus IVF: The Way to Go 27**
Atef Darwish

Chapter 3 **The Use of rLH, HMG and hCG in Controlled Ovarian Stimulation for Assisted Reproductive Technologies 53**
Micah J. Hill and Anthony M. Propst

Chapter 4 **The Means of Progress in Improving the Results of *in vitro* Fertilization Based on the Identification and Correction of the Pathology of Hemostasis 77**
Andrey Momot, Inna Lydina, Lyudmila Tsyvkina, Oksana Borisova and Galina Serdyuk

Chapter 5 **Intracytoplasmic Sperm Injection – Factors Affecting Fertilization 117**
Murid Javed and Essam Michael

Chapter 6 **SubEndometrial Embryo Delivery (SEED) with Egg Donation – Mechanical Embryo Implantation 145**
Michael Kamrava and Mei Yin

Chapter 7 **Luteal Phase Support in ART: An Update 155**
Mohamad E. Ghanem and Laila A. Al-Boghdady

Preface

Since its first description by Steptoe and Edward, IVF gained popularity among both doctors and patients. There is many studies on assisted reproduction and they cover most of the related technical, laboratory as well as clinical aspects. To write a book on assisted reproduction nowadays seems very difficult due to a wide plethora of related papers and well-illustrated books. This small-sized book aims at refinement of some already known points of practical importance in infertility management particularly ART. Before advising couples to start a protocol of ART, gynecologists shouldn't ignore proper preoperative assessment of the female. A lot of money and stress can be eliminated if the patient has a proper combined laparoscopy and hysteroscopy. In this book, an unbiased stratification plan for every infertile case is demonstrated before referring her to ART. The established role of endoscopic preparation for ART is well addressed. Many failures can be prevented when a simple office hysteroscopy is performed before starting the cycle. Moreover, success can be increased by utilizing some assisted endoscopic embryo transfer techniques particularly in cases with recurrent implantation failure.

Induction of superovulation is a subject of debate particularly in poor responders. In this book, you will find that the inclusion of LH in the stimulation of poor responders and women thirty-five and older would improve ART outcomes. If you are an embryologist, you will enjoy reading a detailed chapter on technical updated tricks that would be very valuable in all steps of lab work. For clinicians, a modified technique of embryo transfer as well a detailed discussion of luteal phase support protocols will be address in two separate chapter.

In short, this book is tailored to add new ideas or tricks to different steps of ART. We hope it would serve as a foundation of valuable information to all gynecologists that they all find useful during ART day practice.

Dr. Atef M.M. Darwish, MD, PhD
Department of Obstetrics and Gynecology,
Woman's Health University Hospital,
Egypt

Chapter 1

The Role of Endoscopy in Management of Infertility

Jozsef Daru and Attila Keresztruri

Additional information is available at the end of the chapter

http://dx.doi.org/10.5772/51094

1. Introduction

1.1. Laparoscopy

1.1.1. Methods, techniques and equipment

Laparoscopy is used world-wide to investigate infertility. It is a minimally invasive surgical technique used in infertility diagnosis and treatment and generally accepted that diagnostic laparoscopy is the gold standard in diagnosing tubal pathology and other intra - abdominal causes of infertility. Laparoscopic surgery has revolutionized gynecological surgery. In a female, the uterus, fallopian tubes and ovaries are located in the pelvis which is at the very bottom of the abdomen. Laparoscopy allows seeing abnormalities that might interfere with a woman's ability to conceive a pregnancy. Infertility diagnostic and operative laparoscopy help evaluate gynecological problems such as uterine fibroids, structural abnormalities of the uterus, endometriosis, ovarian cysts and adhesions. A large number of procedures can be performed laparoscopically. Most commonly it is used to inspect the pelvic organs (diagnostic laparoscopy), and often to perform surgical procedures (operative laparoscopy) at the same time. Complicated endometriosis, pelvic adhesions, removal of large ovarian cysts and fibroids should only be performed by highly skilled laparoscopic surgeons. The fiber-optic camera on the laparoscope is very small. It is inserted into the body, through an incision made in the nave, another incision may be made near the upper pubic region.

1.2. Laparoscopy is often used for

- evaluating infertility
- treating the fallopian tubes
- removing scar tissue or adhesions
- treating endometriosis

- removing ovarian cysts
- unexplained infertility
- abnormal vaginal bleeding
- abdominal pain
- frequent miscarriage
- Ovarian drilling

Laparoscopy is performed using general anesthesia. This means that the patient is completely asleep during the entire procedure.

2. Basic equipment for laparoscopy

- Laparoscopic Trolley
- Light Source – Halogen
- High flow CO_2 insufflator
- Television monitor
- Video camera
- Videocassette recorder
- Suction/irrigation system
- Primary trocar, 10–12 mm
- Laparoscope, 10–12 mm
- 1 to 3 secondary trocars, 5 mm
- Biopsy forceps
- Blunt manipulating probe
- Bipolar coagulator
- Monopolar coagulator
- Grasping instruments
- Lasers, CO_2, KTP, Nd:YAG or argon
- Laparoscopic Morcellator
- Laparoscope needle holder
- Clip applicator
- Uterine manipulator
- Myoma Screw
- PCOD Needle
- Port Closutre
- Ring Applicator
- Aspiration Needle
- L-Hook
- Cables, such as Cable-Martin, Cable-2 pin and Cables-L&T
- LigaSure

2.1. Laparoscopic microsurgery

In many situations, laparoscopy provides important and essential information in the management of infertility. It is a minimally invasive surgical procedure that uses a small camera that allows direct visual examination of the pelvic reproductive anatomy. Laparoscopy detects endometriosis, scarring, fallopian tube damage, adhesions, ovarian cysts, fibroids, congenital abnormalities and polycystic ovaries. Laparoscopy allows to see abnormalities that might interfere with a woman's ability to conceive a pregnancy. The most common problems are endometriosis , pelvic adhesions , ovarian cysts and uterine fibroids. Laparoscopy less invasive surgery that traditional surgery; offers a closed internal environment, minimal tissue handling, less tissue trauma and is less adhesiogenic. It gives the desired magnification for microsurgery, Traditional surgery requires making an incision in the abdomen which is several centimeters long. This in turn means that the patient has to spend two to three nights in the hospital. After laparoscopy the patient has one to three smaller incisions. Laparoscopy allows seeing the abdominal organs and sometimes making repairs, without making a larger incision that can require a longer recovery time and hospital stay. Each incision may be one half a centimeter to a full centimeter in length. Most often, patients who have had a laparoscopy will be able to go home the same day as the surgery.

2.2. The benefits of laparoscopy

- More accurate diagnosis.
- No stitches.
- Therapeutic benefit
- Shorter recovery time
- Fewer post-op complications Less scarring.

2.3. Indications for laparoscopic microsurgery

- Tubal anastomosis
- Bowel repair
- Bladder repair
- Ureteric repair
- Microsurgical repair of *myoma*
- Neosalpingostomy
- Tubal anastomosis
- Tubocornual inplantation

2.4. Environmental effects of fertility

Environment represents the totality of physical, chemical, biological and socioeconomic factors or conditions that constitute the external milieu surrounding the human organism. Up to 10% of infertility cannot be explained medically. Female factors in infertility stem from ovulation problems, thyroid irregularities, polycystic ovarian syndrome, and fallopian tube obstruction. Geographic differences may suggest environmental exposures that need investigation. Some toxins , gases can also have an impact on a person's fertility. The basic idea was to go to places in the world where we know that people have high level of exposures to substances that are suspected to cause these effects in fertility. Exploring multi-compound exposures is yet another challenge in environmental epidemiology.

2.5. Stress-related female infertility:

- Psychogenic amenorrhea
- Pseudocyesis
- Chronic anovulation
- anorexia nervosa
- Bulimia
- Menstrual dysfunction
- Early pregnancy loss
- Hyperprolactinrmia and amenorrhea

The following factors increase a woman's risk of infertility:

- age
- stress
- overweight or underweight
- tobacco
- alcohol
- sexually transmitted diseases (STDs)
- health problems that cause hormonal changes
- athletic training
- poor diet

2.6. Toxic effect

- Heavy metals
- Centrally acting drugs
- Environmental pesticides
- Hormones

2.7. HSG versus Chromopertubation

The diagnosis of uterine and/or tubal pathology as causes of female infertility represents a fundamental step in the evaluation of the infertile couple. As a tubal factor is a common cause of infertility, evaluation of the infertile couple should include assessment of the fallopian tubes for patency. Several others diagnostic techniques useful to the clinical evaluation of the uterine cavity and tubal anatomy are: transvaginal sonography (TVS), hysterosalpingography (HSG), hysteroscopy and hydrosonography (HDS) and laparoscopy. In the evaluation of uterine and tubo-peritoneal factors causing infertility, almost all the protocols retain hysterosalpingography (HSG), hysteroscopy and laparoscopy, first choice diagnostic tools. HSG was widespread as a test method before the development of the Echovist®, which made it possible to visualize the fallopian tubes with ultrasound. Laparoscopy provides the most comprehensive information on the status of the internal genitalia. It permits the use of a contrast medium or dye to examine the fallopian tubes (chromopertubation). Secondly, the procedure provides important information regarding the presence of adhesions, inflammatory changes and endometriosis.

2.8. Endometriosis and infertility

Endometriosis is a condition in which endometrium tissue, normally found lining the uterus, spreads to other areas within a woman's pelvic cavity and abdomen, usually the fallopian tubes, ovaries and intestines. It is a leading cause of disability among reproductive age women secondary to infertility and pelvic pain. The epidemiology of endometriosis is poorly defined. The most widely accepted hypothesis is that endometrial cells are transported from the uterine cavity and subsequently become implanted at ectopic sites. Retrograde flow of menstrual tissue through the fallopian tubes could transport endometrial cells intra-abdominally; the lymphatic or circulatory system could transport endometrial cells to distant sites (eg, the pleural cavity). Another hypothesis is coelomic metaplasia: Coelomic epithelium is transformed into endometrium-like glands. According to medical statistics the infertility can affect around 40% of women with Endometriosis. Pelvic examination may be normal, or findings may include a retroverted and fixed uterus, enlarged ovaries, fixed ovarian masses, thickened rectovaginal septum, indurations of the cul-de-sac, and nodules on the uterosacral ligament. Rarely, lesions can be seen on the vulva or cervix or in the vagina, umbilicus, or surgical scars. Association between endometriosis and autoimmune diseases such as rheumatoid arthritis, systemic lupus erythematosus, hypothyroidism, hyperthyroidism, and multiple sclerosis have recently been described. In order to properly diagnose endometriosis, it is necessary to have a laparoscopy performed. During a Laparoscopic procedure, endometrial implants can be easily seen once these implants have reached a reasonable size. Endometriosis may be found in up to 50% of infertile women, according to the American Society for Reproductive Medicine.

The sins of endometriosis

- General Pelvic Pain
- Painful Sexual Intercourse
- Heavy Menstrual Periods
- Infertility
- Bladder Problems
- Constipation and/or Diarrhea
- Family History of Endometriosis

Patophysiology of infertility in endometriotic patients:

- Increased prostaglandin level
- Sperm motility and binding
- Vascular Endothelial Growth Factor (VEGF)
- Tumor Necrosis Factor alpha(TNF-α)
- Immunological abnormalities
- Abnormal follicular development
- Reduced embryo implantation

Some patients with minimal endometriosis and normal pelvic anatomy are also infertile; reasons for impaired fertility include the following:

- Increased incidence of luteinized unruptured ovarian follicle syndrome (trapped oocyte)
- Increased peritoneal prostaglandin production or peritoneal macrophage activity (resulting in oocyte phagocytosis)
- Nonreceptive endometrium (because of luteal phase dysfunction or other abnormalities)

2.9. Endoscopic techniques in endometriosis

Infertility and pelvic pain in its various forms are the main expressions of endometriosis. The fallopian tubes and ovaries may adhere to the lining of the pelvis or to each other, restricting their movement. Another factor which cause infertility with Endometriosis, may be the over-production of prostaglandins. No laboratory findings are particularly helpful in making or confirming a diagnosis of endometriosis. Treatment of endometriosis, medical or surgical, is directed at ameliorating the symptoms and severity of the pelvic pain and infertility. Some of the options for treatment to conceive include:

- Medical therapy(GnRH, danasol,Ru486(Mifepristone),selective estrogen receptor modulators, TNF-α inhibitors,
- Ultrasound-guided aspiration
- Laparoscopic surgery
- IVF treatment
- IUI
- acupuncture
- NSAIDs for discomfort
- Drugs to suppress ovarian function

Surgery may include lysis of adhesions, restoration of normal anatomy and ablation of all endometriotic implants, cystectomy or resection of endometriomas and in extreme cases even the removal of the ovaries and the uterus. During laparoscopy can remove endometrial growths, scar tissue, and adhesions caused by the endometriosis. This is not a really cure, and endometriosis may return later. However, some women will have increased fertility for up to 6- 9 months after surgery.

2.10. Management of endometrioma

Endometriomas usually present as a pelvic mass arising from growth of ectopic endometrial tissue within the ovary. They typically contain thick brown tar-like fluid (hence the name "chocolate cyst"). Ultrasound is useful for supporting the clinical diagnosis of endometrioma. In case of infertility, the management of endometriomas is controversial. Many women with endometriosis can conceive naturally. For those who have difficulty, surgery often provides a "window of opportunity" during which the chances of conception increase the medical treatment alone usually is inadequate. The ultrasound-guided aspiration of the chocolate-colored fluid aspiration sometimes have serious consequences including post aspiration infection, pelvic adhesions, and ovarian abscess. Laparoscopic cystectomy is the gold standard, and preferred approach for the treatment of endometriosis and endometrioma.

Surgical treatment is associated with a high recurrence rate and its employment for women undergoing assisted conception.. Excision of the entire cyst by laparoscopy or laparotomy appears to be the optimum treatment approach. Fenestration and ablation of the lining of an endometrioma is a less preferred option. Aspiration alone is ineffective. Laparoscopic drainage of endometriomas has the same disadvantages as ultrasound-guided aspiration. The recurrence rate is very high (80-90%). Fenestration and ablation is also less effective than excision, both in terms of improving fertility and for reducing pain. Laparoscopic cystectomy remains a first-line choice for the treatment of endometrioma. This consists of: opening the cyst, identifying the cyst wall and removing it from the ovarian cortex by traction and with grasping forceps. Surgery is not only the elimination of the endometrioma effectively but also to reconstruct the pelvic anatomy. The advantage of medical treatment has not been shown to be effective in controlling symptoms or improving fertility potential. After surgical treatment GnRH for a period of 12 weeks or dienogest (Visanne®, 2 mg) should be useful. Birth control pills have been shown to be ineffective in postoperative treatment of endometriomas. Recurrent ovarian surgery is not recommended.

It is generally accepted, that patients with endometriosis have lower success rates with IVF than patients without endometriosis. Several investigations have been occurring to improve the pregnancy rates following treatment with IVF in patients with endometrioma.

2.11. Adhesions - laparoscopic adhesiolysis

Adhesions are bands of scar tissue that connect normally separated pelvic structures. Postoperative adhesions occur in 60% to 90% of patients undergoing major gynecologic surgery. Pelvic adhesions (scars) develop as a normal tissue response to inflammation, which occurs whenever the tissue is damaged. Adhesions are a frequent cause of infertility and pelvic pain in women. Pelvic adhesions impair fertility by disrupting normal tubal-ovarian relationships. Postoperative adhesions are squeal of impaired fibrinolysis of the fibrin and cellular exudates after peritoneal injury. Both microsurgical and laparoscopic techniques are used to treat pelvic adhesions. Additional studies also indicate the benefit of adhesiolysis in treating infertility. The most important factors which suppress fibrinolytic activity and promote adhesion formation are:

- Port wound just above the target of dissection
- Tissue Ischemia
- Prolonged operation
- Visceral injury
- Drying of serosal surfaces
- Blood clots
- Traction of peritoneum
- History of infection in the abdominal cavity
- Endometriosis
- Previous intra-abdominal trauma or bleeding (ectopic pregnancy, motor vehicle accidents, appendicitis)

- Surgical glove powder
- Delayed postoperative mobilization of patient

Causes of pelvic adhesions

- Previous pelvic or abdominal surgery (most common reason)
- History of cancer or radiation therapy

The incidence and severity of adhesions

- no adhesion
- filmy avascular adhesions
- vascular adhesions
- cordlike fibrous adhesions
- plain fibrous adhesions

Prevention of adhesions in surgery

With an optimal surgical technique intending to minimize mesothelial injury, peritoneal trauma is inevitable. laparoscopy leads to less adhesion formation compared to open surgery.

The most commonly used agents for preventing postoperative adhesions:

2.12. Adhesion Prevention Techniques

- Gentle Tissue Handling
- Use of Barrier Agents
- Precise Treatment of the Surgical Area
- Minimal Blood Loss
- Copious Pelvic Irrigation
- No Glove Powder Exposure
- Antibiotics
- Barriers (solid membranes, liquids)
- Antihistamines
- Hormones
- Nonsteroids

2.13. Laparoscopic adhesiolysis

Adhesiolysis is essential to restore normal tubo-ovarian anatomical relationships. The basic principles for carrying out adhesiolysis are followed: If the adhesion is thin and avascular, it is easily lysed and the chances of recurrence are not much. If adhesion is thick and highly vascular it is difficult to separate. Theses adhesion requires use of energy (Unipolar or Bipolar, Ultrasonic dissector). After achieving haemostasis sharp dissection with scissors are necessary. After adhesiolysis some fluid can be left inside to prevent recurrence or high molecular weight dextran tried to prevent re-adhesion. The fertility results after adhesiolysis are correlated with the state of the adhesions.

2.14. Complications

The most common intraoperative complication is injury to the bowel. With dense adhesions, this risk increases. Other intraoperative complications may include bleeding and injury to adjacent organs such as the gallbladder, spleen, ovaries, especially when working next to these organs-

3. Myomectomy

Uterine fibroids are the most common pelvic tumor, occurring in about 70% of women by age 45. However, many fibroids are small and asymptomatic. About 25% of white and 50% of black women have symptomatic fibroids. Fibroids are benign tumors of the muscle of the uterus most myomas do not cause clinical symptoms and do not require intervention. Based on location the various types of myoma are subserous, intramural and submucous fibroid. Most frequently, they develop in the myometrial wall and can lead to uterine distortion. Common problems associated with myomas are pelvic, abdominal, or back discomfort; urinary bladder irritability; abnormal uterine bleeding; bowel dysfunction; infertility; and pregnancy loss and/or complications. Myomas can cause infertility are mechanical interference with implantation, sperm and embryo transport, focal endometrial vascular and endocrine disturbances, endometrial inflammation, and abnormal uterine contractility. During the past few years, there have been a number of studies advancing the knowledge about the efficacy and safety of treatments of myomas, including medical and minimally invasive therapies. Laparoscopic myomectomy was first described by Semm and Metler in 1980 for subserosal fibroid there is an increasing trend for minimal access surgery for treatment of uterine myomas. Laparoscopic myomectomy is a very recent advance in the field of gynaecological surgery. Laparoscopic myomectomy has provided minimal invasive alternative to laparotomy with advantage of faster recovery and less postoperative adhesions. Laparoscopic myomectomy (LM) is an effective technique that is associated with the development of operative laparoscopic equipment and surgical techniques. The size does not matter for performance of a myomectomy laparoscopically. Laparoscopic myomectomy has evolved into a safe, efficient, and cost effective approach for the treatment of intramural, subserosal, and pedunculated fibroids. Criteria for myomectomy for surgical intervention, supported by the American College of Obstetricians and Gynecologists (ACOG) and American society for reproductive medicine (ASRM) are:

- Clinically apparent myomas that are a significant concern to the patient even if otherwise asymptomatic;
- Myomas causing excessive bleeding and/or anemia;
- Myomas causing acute or chronic pain; and
- Myomas causing significant urinary problems not due to other abnormalities;
- Infertility with distortion of the endometrial cavity or tubal occlusion.

Before myomectomy, Hysteroscopy is performed in most patients at the outset of the procedure, than all pelvic structures and the abdominal cavity are inspected

Steps of operation: subserosal myomas

- Injection with vasopressin.
- Positioning of Roeder loop around the base of the myoma.
- Coagulation of the capsule.
- Incision of the capsule.
- Myoma enucleation.
- Tension on the Roeder loop.
- Dissection of myoma.
- Closure of the capsule with Roeder loop or linear stapler.
- Myoma extraction with Morcellator.

Steps of operation: intramural and deep subserosal myomas

- Injection with vasopressin.
- Regulation of entry point for incision.
- Incision of uterus and capsule.
- Enucleation of myoma.
- Dislocation of myoma
- Coagulation of uterine bed.
- Closure of wound with deep muscular and superficial serosal closure.
- Morcellator and extraction of myoma.

3.1. Complications

- Secondary hemorrhage may occur
- Gastrointestinal injuries
- Adhesions
- Inflammations

3.2. Modalities of laparoscopic myomectomy

- Laparoscopic assisted myomectomy (LAM)
- Laparoscopic assisted Trans vaginal myomectomy
- Robotic laparoscopic myomectomy
- Laparoscopic myolysis and cryosurgery

Laparoscopic myomectomy generally is associated with shorter hospitalization; laparoscopic myomectomy is a benefit when traditional surgical management and future fertility are declined. After myomectomy the conception rate is approximately 53-70%. Laparoscopic uterine surgery predisposes an increased risk of uterine rupture during pregnancy, and delivery.

3.3. Infertility and Polycystic Ovary Syndrome

Polycystic ovarian syndrome (PCOS) is a fairly common condition. The incidence of Polycystic ovarian syndrome (PCOS) varies between 3% and 15% of women of reproductive age, depending on the population studied and the diagnostic criteria applied. The cause of PCOS is unknown. However, PCOS is thought to be a genetic disorder (autosomal dominant) meaning that each child has a 50% chance of inheriting the disorder from a parent who carries the gene. The gene can be inherited from either mother or father. The exact gene causing PCOS has not yet been identified. The condition was first described in 1935 by American gynecologists Irving F. Stein, Sr. and Michael L. Leventhal, from whom its original name of *Stein-Leventhal syndrome* is taken.

In 1990 a consensus workshop sponsored by the NIH/NICHD suggested that a patient has PCOS if she has all of the following:

1. oligoovulation
2. signs of androgen excess (clinical or biochemical)
3. other entities are excluded that would cause polycystic ovaries

In 2003 a consensus workshop sponsored by ESHRE/ASRM in Rotterdam indicated PCOS to be present if any 2 out of 3 criteria are met

1. oligoovulation and/or anovulation
2. excess androgen activity
3. polycystic ovaries (by gynecologic ultrasound)

The insulin resistance with compensatory hyperinsulinemia is e prominent feature of the syndrome and seems to have a pathophysiologic role in the hyperanrogenism. It is a common hormonal disorder that is poorly understood and clinically characterized by lack of regular ovulation, irregular menstrual cycles, infertility, abnormal facial hair growth, obesity and polycystic ovaries. Polycystic ovarian syndrome can be difficult to diagnose because not all patients with PCOS display the same symptoms. Polycystic ovarian syndrome is a disorder characterized by insulin resistance and a compensatory elevated insulin level, which are found in both the overweight and non-overweight woman with the syndrome. In addition the patients has a risk for possible long-term metabolic hazards such as Type 2 diabetes mellitus, dyslipidemia, and cardiovascular disease. The symptoms of PCOS and their severity can vary from patient to patient;

- Irregular, absent, or few menstrual cycles
- Infertility
- Elevated levels of insulin, resistance to insulin, or diabetes
- Multiple cysts on ovaries
- Enlarged ovaries
- Obesity concentrated in the midsection
- Acne or oily skin
- High blood pressure
- Excess facial or body hair
- Thinning hair on the scalp

3.4. Standard diagnostic assessments

- History-taking, specifically for menstrual pattern, obesity, hirsutism, and the absence of breast development.
- Gynecologic ultrasonography, specifically looking for small ovarian follicles
- Serum (blood) levels of androgens, sex hormone-binding globulin (SHBG), LH (Luteinizing hormone), FSH (Follicle stimulating hormone),estrogen, and progesterone
- Fasting biochemical screen and lipid profile
- 2-hour oral glucose tolerance test (GTT)
- Laparoscopic examination

3.5. Differential diagnosis

Other causes of irregular or absent menstruation and hirsutism, such as:

- Hypothyroidism,
- Congenital adrenal hyperplasia (21-hydroxylase deficiency),
- Cushing's syndrome,
- Hyperprolactinemia,
- Androgen secreting neoplasmas, and
- Other pituitary or adrenal disorders

PCOS has been reported in other insulin-resistant situations such as acromegaly

3.6. Therapy

Diet: Where PCOS is associated with overweight or obesity, successful weight loss is the most effective method of restoring normal ovulation/menstruation

Exercise

3.7. Symptomatic treatments

Anti-Androgens: Spironolactone (Aldactone), Cyproterone acetate, Flutamide (Eulexin), Finasteride (Propecia, Proscar)

Anti-Obesity Drugs: Orlistat (Xenical), Sibutramine (Meridia)

Metformin: National Institute for Health and Clinical Excellence recommended in 2004 that women with PCOS and a body mass index above 25 be given metformin when other therapy has failed to produce results. Metformin treatment reduces hyperinsulinemia, LH levels, free testosterone concentrations, in overweight women with PCOs. Metformin improves menstrual cyclicity and increases the frequency of ovulation.

Clomiphene citrate (Clomid, Serophene) alone or in combination with weigh loss can be used to induce ovulation or with other, more aggressive, treatments for infertility. Including injection of gonadotropin hormones and assisted reproductive technologies may also be required in women who desire pregnancy and do not become pregnant on Clomid therapy (Gonadotropin injections, hCG , human chorionic gonadotropin, GnRH Lutrepulse).The primary indications for the use of CC is normogonadotropic normoprolactinemic anovulatory infertility i.e. PCOS. Approximately 70-80% of the women will ovulate half of which will conceive.

IVF (in-vitro fertilization)

Steroid hormones: Oral contraceptives (birth control pills), Progesterone (bioidentical), Estrogens, and Corticosteroids

Bilateral wedge resection of ovaries were abandoned due to peri - ovarian adhesion formation.

Ovarian drilling: Surgical procedure which can help induce ovulation in some women who have not responded to other treatments for PCOS. In this procedure a small portion of ovarian tissue is destroyed by an electric current delivered through a needle inserted into the ovary. This is less invasive technique and less chances of multiple Pregnancy and ovarian hyperstimulation. Laparoscopic Ovarian Drilling is a safe and cost effective procedure and increases the sensitivity to gonadotrophins.

Tubal factor

Physiology of the fallopian tube

The fallopian tube has complex task:

- Pick up the released ovum
    - Transport the spermatozoa towards the ampulla
    - Sperm activation
    - Fertilization support
    - Embryo cleavage
    - Zygote transport

Tubal infertility includes the changes due to inflammation which affect the fallopian tube and its relation towards the ovary in a way that will affect ovulation, the transport of the egg, sperm, or embryo, or alter the function of the tube as the site of fertilization. Injury the distal oviduct resulting in a complete or partial occlusion is the most common tubal lesion. Microsurgical or laparoscopic repair is the primary method of treatment with pregnancy rates. Hydrosalpinges produces an adverse impact on results of *in vitro* fertilization. Removal of Hydrosalpinges will improve IVF success rates. The surgeon has to distinguish between the pathological findings according to the site which is affected.

This are:

1. Distal tubal obstruction (complete or incomplete)
2. Hydrosalpinx.
3. Isthmo-cornual block (complete or incomplete).
4. Any combination of the previous three categories.
5. Peritubal or periovarian adhesions.

3.8. Reversal of sterilization

Laparoscopic surgery offers greater comfort to the patients and is more economical, with shorter operative and postoperative hospitalization than laparotomy. Laparoscopic procedures limit the risk of postoperative adhesions to. Operative laparoscopy may be an alternative to microsurgery by laparotomy for management of tubal lesions. Many people, including doctors, mistakenly believe that tubal sterilization is permanent and irreversible. Tubal reversal surgery can also be performed laparoscopically. The laparoscopic technique uses magnification and allows much less pain, discomfort, disfigurement and adhesion formation than the traditional open method. Because the laparoscopic approach to tubal ligation reversal surgery is relatively new technique there is a limited amount of experience worldwide. Tubal ligation is performed for birth control. Tubal ligation blocks the fallopian tubes preventing the egg and sperm from passing through the fallopian tubes. Procedures are performed in several different ways including: burning, removal of a piece, placement of a tight surgical band or clip on the fallopian tube. People sometimes change their minds. The removal of this blockage is the tubal reversal. Tubal reanastomosis surgically opens the fallopian tubes to allow the sperm to reach the egg. When the tubes are severely damaged IVF is the first choice. A laparoscopic approach may be recommended especially in overweight patients where the abdominal wall is too thick to do the procedure the more common way by minilaparotomy. Laparoscopy allows the surgeon to inspect the tubes first to see if the reanastomosis can be done. The success of reversal is dependent on the amount of fallopian tube that has been damaged. Some tubes do not work well because of the surgery to block them followed by surgery to reopen them. In other circumstances a woman's age or her husband's sperm count are preventing success following tubal reversal surgery. Tubal reversal has a higher risk of ectopic pregnancy. Tubal reversal surgery is same-day surgery and takes between two and four weeks to recover. The success rate is greater than 75% for pregnancy.

3.9. Tubal reversal surgeries:

- Tubo - tubal anastomosis
- Tubo - uterine implantation
- Ampullary salpingostomy
- Mini-laparotomy tubal reversal
- Laparoscopic tubal reversal
- Robotic assisted tubal reversal
- Essure sterilization reversal
- Adiana sterilization reversal

Tubal reversal success rates vary widely depending upon many factors. These include the women's ages, methods of tubal ligation that they had performed experience of the surgeon and techniques for repairing the tubes, length of follow-up after reversal surgery among other factors.

4. Salpingitis Isthmica Nodosa

The etiology of salpingitis isthmica nodosa is unknown; however it may be a post infectious reaction. Patients have histological evidence of previous salpingitis and may have high serum Chlamydia antibody titers. The radiological prevalence of SIN is 3.9-7.5%. The disease is usually bilateral (over 50% of cases). In severe cases, it leads to complete obliteration of the tubal lumen. SIN is associated with infertility and ectopic pregnancy. Salpingitis isthmica nodosa is also referred to as tubal diverticulosis. HSG demonstrates multiple small diverticular collections of contrast protruding from the lumen into the wall of the isthmic portion of the fallopian tubes. Histologicaly, the up to 2 mm sized diverticula represent hypertrophied tubal mucosa that penetrates the myosalpinx. There is secondary hyperplasia and hypertrophy of the surrounding myosalpinx, and hence at laparoscopy, localized nodular thickening or swelling of the isthmus is identified.

Laparoscopic finding: enlargement of the tubocornual or isthmic portion of the fallopian tube. The condition is associated with infertility and the occurrence of ectopic pregnancy. The appropriate management of the patients with SIN segmental resection with microtubal reanastomosis.

4.1. Salpingectomy in IVF patients with tubal infertility and hydrosalpinges

Hydrosalpinges are dilated and occluded fallopian tubes generally the result of a prior pelvic infection. These are a cause of female infertility in a number of patients IVF the only option for having a child. The accepted theory today is that the hydrosalpinx fluid plays a causative role in the reduced pregnancy rate with ART. Hydrosalpinx fluid may reduce the receptive ability of the endometrium. It is well known that the success of ART for patients with tubal disease with hydrosalpinx is reduced by half compared with patients without hydrosalpinx. A number of studies were published examining the effect of salpingectomy on IVF pregnancy rates. Removing a hydrosalpinx by laparoscopic salpingectomy may to improve pregnancy rates. Surgical treatment should be considered for all women with hydrosalpinges prior to IVF treatment. In cases of sonographically apparent hydrosalpinges, a salpingectomy, rather than a salpingostomy, is the preferred route of treatment. Some couples, however, may prefer a salpingostomy, which offers some potential of a spontaneous pregnancy, but laparoscopic salpingectomy of hydrosalpinges prior to IVF treatment increases the odds of pregnancy and live birth compared to no treatment.

4.2. Management of ectopic pregnancy

Ectopic pregnancy is a high-risk condition that occurs in 1.9 percent of reported pregnancies. The etiology of ectopic pregnancy remains uncertain although a number of risk factors have been identified. Risk factors most strongly associated with ectopic pregnancy include previous ectopic pregnancy, tubal surgery, assisted reproductive technology, genital infection and pelvic inflammatory disease intrauterine contraceptive device. A history of genital infections or infertility and current smoking increase risk.

4.3. Diagnosis

- Diagnostic tests for ectopic pregnancy include a urine pregnancy test
- Ultrasonography
- beta-hCG measurement
- Occasionally, diagnostic curettage.
- some physicians have used serum progesterone levels
- no combination of physical examination findings can reliably exclude ectopic pregnancy
- 40 percent in a patient with abdominal pain and vaginal bleeding but no other risk factors
- 30 percent of patients with ectopic pregnancies have no vaginal bleeding
- 10 percent have a palpable adnexal mass
- 10 percent have negative pelvic examinations
- In cases where an ectopic pregnancy is suspected and ultrasound is inconclusive, a diagnostic laparoscopy may be required.

4.4. Differential diagnosis of ectopic pregnancy

- Acute appendicitis
- Ovarian torsion
- Pelvic inflammatory disease
- Miscarriage
- Ruptured corpus luteum cyst or follicle
- Tubo-ovarian abscess
- Urinary calculi

4.5. Treatment

Expectant management

Is between 47 and 82 percent effective in managing ectopic pregnancy

Medical treatment

Methotrexate, a folic acid antagonist, is a well-studied medical therapy. Side effects of methotrexate include bone marrow suppression, elevated liver enzymes, rash, alopecia, stomatitis, nausea, and diarrhea. The time to resolution of the ectopic pregnancy is three to seven weeks after methotrexate therapy.

Surgical treatment

A laparoscopic approach is preferable to an open approach in a patient who is haemodynamically stable. If the contra lateral tube is healthy, the preferred option is salpingectomy, where the entire Fallopian tube, or the affected segment containing the ectopic gestation, is removed In the pat few years laparoscopy with salpingostomy, without fallopian tube removal, has become the preferred method of surgical treatment. Laparoscopy has similar tubal patency and future fertility rates as medical treatment.

Follow-up and prognosis

During treatment, physicians should examine patients at least weekly and sometimes daily. Serial beta-hCG measurements should be taken after treatment until the level is undetectable.

Adnexal mass in infertility

There are a number of possible disorders that can cause a pelvic mass. Some are common, while others are quite unusual or even rare. The physical exam should include visualization and palpation of the abdomen. The next step is usually an imaging study, such as ultrasound, CAT scan, or MRI

Differential diagnoses

- Uterine fibroids
- Uterine cancer
- Benign ovarian cyst
- Ectopic pregnancy
- Fallopian tube cyst
- Hydrosalpinx
- Ovarian cancer

Follicular cysts

There are several different types of ovarian cysts, the most common being functional cysts. Often, ovarian cysts do not cause symptoms. Women in the age group of thirty to sixty are more prone to having ovarian cysts.The follicular cysts are easily identified on vaginal sonography, usually measure a few millimeters to a few centimeters in size, and rarely become symptomatic. If they enlarge in size they may rupture, producing transient abdominal pain. Ovarian cysts can cause several other problems if they twist, bleed, or rupture

Dermoid cyst

Ovarian dermoid cyst, also known as mature teratoma, is a non cancerous ovarian tumor, which is more commonly found in young women. Although dermoids are non cancerous, in some rare cases, they might develop into cancerous growth. Dermoid cysts may contain substances such as nails and dental, cartilage like, and bonelike structures. These growths can develop in a woman during her reproductive years. Dermoids can range in size anywhere between two to ten centimeters. It is very difficult to identify the presence of these cysts inside the ovaries as they do not produce any symptoms. They can cause torsion, infection, rupture, and cancer. These dermoid cysts can be removed with either conventional surgery or laparoscopy. Ovarian dermoid cysts do not affect the fertility of the woman.

Tubo ovarian abscess

Tubo-ovarian abscess is an advanced form of pelvic inflammatory disease most often caused by spread of bacteria from the lower genital tract. It is one of the most severe complications of PID and can lead to significant morbidity and occasional mortality. The microbial etiology of TOAs typically is polymicrobial with a mixture of anaerobic, aerobic, and facultative organisms being isolated. The most common bacterial pathogens are anaerobic. Sexually transmitted disease, early age of first sexual encounter, multiple sexual partners, douching, IUDs are at increased risk for pelvic inflammatory disease and tubo-ovarian abscess. Diverticulitis and appendicitis are also potential causes.

5. Differential diagnosis

- Hemorrhagic cyst
- Endometrioma
- Ectopic pregnancy - if pregnancy test positive
- Cystadenoma
- Cystadenocarcinoma
- Dermoid cyst
- Acute appendicitis
- Diverticulitis

5.1. Complications:

Infertility due to tubal occlusion, increased risk of ectopic pregnancy, and chronic pelvic pain as the result of adhesions.

5.2. Therapy

Treatment of TOA historically was surgical with most women having a total abdominal hysterectomy and bilateral salpingo-oophorectomy Management of TOAs has changed drastically in the past decades with the advent of broad-spectrum antibiotics (ampicillin, clindamycin, and flagyl) and continues to evolve with improved imaging and drainage techniques. Recently antibiotics, surgical intervention, with either conventional surgery or laparoscopy to be in use.

Adnexal torsion

Adnexal torsion is an uncommon gynecologic emergency that is caused by the twisting of the ovary, fallopian tube, or both along the vascular pedicle. It is a rare gynecologic emergency of women at reproductive ages. Usually adnexal torsion is a process of benign tumors. The clinical presentation is often nonspecific with few distinctive physical findings, commonly resulting in delay in diagnosis and surgical management. The causes of adnexal torsion include functional and pathologic ovarian cysts, paraovarian cysts, ovarian hyper stimulation, adhesions, ectopic pregnancy, and congenital malformations. Classically, patients present with sudden onset, severe, unilateral lower abdominal pain that worsens intermittently over many hours. Nausea and vomiting occur in approximately 70% of patients, mimicking a gastrointestinal source of pain and further obscuring the diagnosis. Colored Doppler sonography with its non-invasive modality detects blood flow patterns within the ovarian vascular networks and gives important information about the diagnosis of torsion. Laparoscopy surgery must be the choice for less post operative morbidity, and a better cosmetic appearance. Detorsion must be performed even in necrotic appearing adnexa because of a high rate of survival of ovaries even looking necrotic. Salpingo-oophorectomy may be indicated if severe vascular compromise, peritonitis, or tissue necrosis is clearly evident.

6. Endoscopy complications

Diagnostic laparoscopy is normally the standard procedure performed as the final test in the infertility work up before progressing to infertility treatment. For the most part, the risks associated with laparoscopy are of the same type that occurs with traditional surgery. Problems from anesthesia, bleeding and infections can occur with either type of surgery. The risk of damage to internal organs is also possible with either type of surgery. The risks of laparoscopy are minimal. Complications among young, healthy women undergoing laparoscopy are rare and occur only in about three out of 1000 cases. These complications can include injuries to structures in the abdomen such as: injury to the bowel, stomach, urinary bladder, ureters, abdominal and pelvic blood vessels, ovaries and uterus. For such injuries, a laparotomy might be necessary to stop bleeding or make repairs. Most often, these injuries occur when the laparoscope is placed through the navel. The risk of a serious complication is less than 1%. Any surgery can have an anesthesia-related complication or be associated with post-operative infection, Fortunately, all of these complications are very unusual. According to the American Society of Reproductive Medicine, one or two women out of every 100 may develop a complication, usually a minor one. Some common complications include:

- damage to the bladder, bowel, and kidneys
- damage to the blood vessels
- internal bleeding
- infection
- reaction to anesthesia
- bladder infection after surgery
- skin irritation around the areas of incision
- formation of adhesions
- hematomas of the abdominal wall
- infection
- allergic reaction
- nerve damage
- urinary retention
- Weeping Peritoneum

- Gas Embolism
- Blood clots
- Hernia
- Thermal Injury
- Port site metastasis
- Other general anesthesia complications
- Death (around 3 in every 100,000)

Certain conditions make laparoscopic surgery a bad choice. Some of these conditions include:

- Severe congestive heart failure
- Respiratory insufficiency
- Presence of a distended bowel
- Previous laparotomy incisions
- Patients with cardiac disease or COPD
- Patients with numerous previous abdominal surgery
- Old age
- Obesity

As in all aspects of medicine, laparoscopic surgery requires experience on the part of the surgeon in order to afford patients the best possible outcome. Accurate diagnosis and appropriate management of complications are requisite of all surgeons.

7. Hysteroscopy

Hysteroscopy is the visual examination of the canal of the cervix and interior of the uterus.. The device is inserted through the vagina.Using fiber optic technology, the hysteroscope transmits an image of the uterine canal and cavity to a monitor, allowing to properly guide the instrument into the endometrial cavity. Hysteroscopy may be performed in women who have an abnormal uterine bleeding, abnormal Pap test, or postmenopausal bleeding. It may be used to help diagnose causes of infertility or repeated miscarriages. Hysteroscopy may also be used to evaluate polyps, uterine adhesions (Asherman's syndrome), and fibroids, and to locate and remove displaced intrauterine devices (IUDs). There are two types of hysteroscopy. Diagnostic hysteroscopy is performed to examine the uterus for signs of normalcy or abnormality, while operative hysteroscopy is performed to treat a disorder after it has been diagnosed. The procedure is very similar to diagnostic hysteroscopy except that operating instruments such as scissors, biopsy forceps, electocautery instruments, and graspers can be placed into the uterine cavity through a channel in the operative hysteroscope. Hysteroscopy can take from two to five minutes to more than one hour. During hysteroscopy either fluids or CO_2 gas is introduced to expand the cavity.

7.1. Indications

- Asherman's syndrome
- Endometrial polyp
- Gynecologic bleeding

- Endometrial ablation
- Myomectomy for uterine fibroids
- Congenital Uterine malformations
- Evacuation of retained products of conception
- Removal of embedded IUDs
- Infertility:
- sterilization
- Absent/ scanty menses.
- Cornual block.

7.2. The advantages of hysteroscopy

- No incisions
- Shortened hospital stay
- Reduced post-operative pain
- Shortened Convalescence
- Reduced risk of infection
- High patient satisfaction

7.3. Resection of polyps/fibroid

In the past, the treatment of benign uterine lesions metrorrhagia; Hysteroscopic surgery is effective to treat menorrhagia and leiomyomas, and other lesions, such as septate uterus and synechiae. In the last 20 years there has been an increased acceptance of hysteroscopic surgery into the gynecological surgery. Diagnostic hysteroscopy is a highly sensitive and specific technique for the management of uterine bleeding problems. It may distinguish between myomas or polyps and provides additional information about surrounding endometrium. Endometrial polyp is the commonest pathology among the structural uterine abnormalities. A polyp is attached to the intestinal wall either by a stalk, peduncles, or by a broad base. The sizes of uterine polyps range from a few millimeters — no larger than a sesame seed — to several centimeters — golf ball sized or larger. Many women with myomata, polyps, uterine septae, and synechiae may now benefit from the convenience of hysteroscopic therapy compared to more aggressive surgical techniques. Hysteroscopy is the first choice in the resection for the treatment of endometrial polyps in women with abnormal uterine bleeding and postmenopausal metrorrhagia. The greatest advantage of hysteroscopic myomectomy is the quick recovery time. The prevalence of malignancy or atypical hyperplasia is 3.2% in women with symptoms and 3.9% in those without symptoms. Transcervical resection is the gold standard for treatment of endometrial polyps. Uterine polyps most commonly occur in women in their 40s and 50s.

7.4. Intrauterine adhesions- adhesiolysis

Intrauterine adhesions develop as a result of intrauterine trauma. Intrauterine adhesions can be asymptomatic and of no clinical significance. Symptoms associated with clinically significant intrauterine adhesions include:

- Infertility
- Menstrual irregularities (hypomenorrhea, amenorrhea)
- Cyclic pelvic pain
- Recurrent pregnancy loss.

The diagnosis is based upon visualization of intrauterine adhesions either directly by hysteroscopy, or indirectly by imaging. The standard treatment of intrauterine adhesions is surgery with lysis under direct visualization. Intrauterine adhesions are cut hysteroscopically using current so that the uterine cavity appears normal. This is usually performed as an ambulatory procedure using operative hysteroscopy. Postoperative management is focused upon reducing the risk of reformation of adhesions.

7.5. Septum resection

Complete septum extending from fundus of uterus till cervix. Hysteroscopic resection uses hysteroscopy to operate within the uterine cavity. An intrauterine septum is cut using current, so that the uterine cavity becomes normal. Polyps, fibroids and uterine septums may be treated with this technique.

7.6. Hysteroscopic resection of fibroid

A local or general anesthetic may be used. The uterus is filled with fluid and the hysteroscope is inserted through the cervix into the uterus. This device guides the physician to the fibroid, which is then removed in pieces with a wire loop. Sometimes a second procedure is needed to remove the entire fibroid. Pregnancy rates have been high among women who had this procedure to remove a fibroid that was causing fertility problems.

7.7. Hysteroscopic metroplasty

Congenital uterine malformations are a group of miscellaneous anomalies in the uterine cavity that may alter the reproductive outcome of the patient. Each type of uterine anomaly has a different impact on pregnancy outcome. These are usually asymptomatic, but are sometimes associated with recurrent pregnancy loss or infertility. A uterine septum is a fibrous band that divides an otherwise normal womb into two halves. It is a much commoner condition than bicornuate uterus and can be associated with subfertility or recurrent miscarriage Obstetrical prognosis of patients presenting repeated pregnancy loss and septate uterus is statistically improved by hysteroscopic metroplasty. Hysteroscopic metroplasty is a day-case procedure and pregnancy can be attempted soon afterwards.

7.8. Office hysteroscopy

There have been a number of studies published that indicates office-based hysteroscopy identifies uterine defects in a large number of infertility patients. Office hysteroscopy is a very simple procedure that requires minimal instrumentation. Office hysteroscopy is advantageous both to the patient and the physician. Office-based hysteroscopy has many benefits to diagnose and treat uterine defects which should improve embryo implantation and pregnancy rates. Hysteroscopy can be performed in a routine office exam room. Office hysteroscopy has been performed using carbon dioxide. Diagnostic office hysteroscopy is a safe procedure, with few significant complications, and the patient can resume normal activities immediately.

7.9. Complications

Complications occur rarely during hysteroscopy A possible problem is uterine perforation when either the hysteroscope itself or one of its operative instruments breaches the wall of the uterus. Injury of the bowel during a perforation, the resulting peritonitis can be fatal. Cervical laceration, intrauterine infection, electrical and laser injuries, and complications caused by the distention media can be frequently encountered. The use of insufflations media can lead to serious and even fatal complications due to embolism or fluid overload with electrolyte imbalances. Other possible complications include allergic reactions and bleeding. The overall complication rate for diagnostic and operative hysteroscopy is 2% with serious complications occurring in less than 1% of cases. The complications of hysteroscopy:

- Bleeding
- Infection
- Perforation of the uterus (rare)/damage to cervix
- Pelvic inflammatory disease
- Complications from fluid or gas used to expand the uterus

Author details

Jozsef Daru and Attila Kereszturi
Department of Obstetrics and Gynecology, University of Szeged, Hungary

8. References

American Association of Clinical Endocrinologists. American Association of Clinical Endocrinologists position statement on metabolic and cardiovascular consequences of polycystic ovary syndrome. National Guideline Clearinghouse. Accessed August 28, 2009.

Barnhart KT, Gosman G, Ashby R, Sammel M. The medical management of ectopic pregnancy: a meta-analysis comparing "single dose" and "multidose" regimens. *Obstet Gynecol*. 2003;101:778–84.

Bhatla N, Dash BB, Kriplani A, Agarwal N. (2009). "Myomectomy during pregnancy: a feasible option.". *J Obstet Gynaecol Res. 2009 Feb;35(1):173-5.*

Bradley LD. Uterine fibroid embolization: a viable alternative to hysterectomy. *AJOG*. 2009 August. 127-135.

Bulun SE. Endometriosis. *N Engl J Med*. 2009 Jan 15;360(3):268-79

Caspi B, Levi R, Appelman Z et al. Conservative management of ovarian cystic teratoma during pregnancy and labor. Am J Obstet Gynecol 182:503-5, 2000

Consensus on infertility treatment related to polycystic ovary syndrome. *Fertil Steril*. Mar 2008;89(3):505-22.

Dharia Patel SP, Steinkampf MP, Whitten SJ, Malizia BA. Robotic Tubal Anastomosis: Surgical Technique and Cost Effectiveness. Fertil Steril. 2008 (4):1175-9

Hegde A, Sinha R. Comment on: Safe entry techniques during laparoscopy: Left upper quadrant entry using the ninth intercostal space-a review of 918 procedures. J Minim Invasive Gynecol 2005;12:463-5

Heinonen PK. Complete septate uterus with longitudinal vaginal septum. *Fertil Steril*. 2006;85:700-705.

Jansen FW, Kolkman W, Bakkum EA, et al. Complications of laparoscopy: an inquiry about closed- versus open-entry technique. Am J Obstet Gynecol 2004; 190:634.

Jones K.D.,Fan A, et al:The ovarian endometrioma; why it is so poorly managed, Hum.Reprod. 2002; 17,845-849

K. Bancroft, C. A. Vaughan Williams, M. Elstein. Pituitary–ovarian function in women with minimal or mild endometriosis and otherwise unexplained infertility. Clinical Endocrinology Volume 36 Issue 2,2008.

Lieng M, Istre O, Qvigstad E. Treatment of endometrial polyps: a systematic review. Acta Obstetricia et Gynecologica Scandinavica.2010;89(8):992-1002

Metter L, Hucke J, Bojahr B, Tinneberg HR, Leyland B, Avelar R. A safety and efficacy study of a resorbable hydrogel for reduction of post-operative adhesions following myomectomy. *Hum Reprod*. 2008. 23(5):1093-1100.

Mismer S.A.,Cramer D.W:The epidemiology of endometriosis. Obstet.Gynecol. Clin.North.Am. 2003; 30:1-19

Murdoch, J. A., and T. J. Gan. "Anesthesia for Hysteroscopy." *Anesthesiology Clinics of North America* 19, no. 1 (March 2001): 125–40.

Ness RB, Trautmann G, Richter HE, et al. Effectiveness of treatment strategies of some

Nezhat C, Kimberly K, Iatrogenic myomas: A new class of myomas. J Min Inv Gynecol 2010;17:544-50.

Nezhat C, Lavie O, Hsu S, Watson J, Barnett O, Lemyre M. Robotic-assisted laparoscopic myomectomy compared with standard laparoscopic myomectomy-a retrospective matched control study. *Fertil Steril*. 2008 Mar 28.

Nouri K, Ott J, Huber JC, Fischer EM, Stogbauer L, Tempfer CB. (2010). "Reproductive outcome after hysteroscopic septoplasty in patients with septate uterus - a retrospective cohort study and systematic review of the literature". *Reprod Biol Endocrinol. 2010 May 21;8(1):52*

Nur MM, Newman IM, Siqueira LM. Glucose metabolism in overweight Hispanic adolescents with and without polycystic ovary syndrome. *Pediatrics.* Sep 2009;124(3):e496-502.

Onders RP, Mittendorf EA. Utility of laparoscopy in chronic abdominal pain. *Surgery.* 2003;134(4):549-552.

Pabuccu R, Gomel V. Reproductive outcome after hysteroscopic metroplasty in women with septate uterus and otherwise unexplained infertility. Fertil Steril 2004;81:1675- 8.

Palomba S, Falbo A, Russo T, Rivoli L, Orio M, Cosco AG, et al. The risk of a persistent glucose metabolism impairment after gestational diabetes mellitus is increased in patients with polycystic ovary syndrome. *Diabetes Care.* Apr 2012;35(4):861-7.

PCOS Consensus Workshop Group. Rotterdam ESHRE/ASRM-Sponsored PCOS Consensus Workshop Group. Revised 2003 consensus on diagnostic criteria and long-term health risks related to polycystic ovary syndrome. *Fertil Steril.* Jan 2004;81(1):19-25

Polena, V., et al. "Long-term results of hysteroscopic myomectomy in 235 patients." *European Journal of Obstetrics & Gynecology and Reproductive Biology* 130 (2007): 232-237.

Reissman P, Spira RM. Laparoscopy for adhesions. *Semin Laparopsc Surg.* 2004;10(4):185-190.

Rodgers AK, Goldberg JM, Hammel JP, Falcone T. Tubal Anastomosis By Robotic Compared With Outpatient Minilaparotomy. Obstet Gynecol. 2007 (6):1375-80

Rossetti A, Sizzi O, Soranna L, Cucinelli F, Mancuso S, Lanzone A. Long-term results of laparoscopic myome-ctomy: recurrence rate in comparison with abdominal myomectomy.Hum Reprod 2001;16(4):770-4

Salim S. Won H. Nesbitt-Hawes E. Campbell N. Abbott J. Diagnosis and management of endometrial polyps: a critical review of the literature. Journal of Minimally Invasive Gynecology. 18(5):569-81

Shakiba K, Bena JF, McGill KM, Minger J, Falcone T. Surgical treatment of endometriosis: a 7-year follow-up on the requirement for further surgery. *Obstet Gynecol.* 2008 Jun;111(6):1285-92

Sinha R, Sundaram M. Laparoscopic management of large myomas. J Gynecol Endosc Surg 2009;1:73-82.

Stewart EA, Rabinovici J, Tempany CM, Inbar Y, Regan L, Gostuot B, et al. Clinical outcomes of focused ultrasound surgery for the treatment of uterine fibroids. *Fertil Steril.* 2006;85:22-29.

Strandell A The influence of hydrosalpinx on IVF and embrio transfer:a review-Hum.Reprod. Update 2000;6:387-395

Swank DJ, Swank-Bordewijk SC, Hop WC, et al. Laparoscopic adhesiolysis in patients with chronic abdominal pain: a blinded randomized controlled multi-center trial. *Lancet.* 2003;361(9536):1247-1251.

Thomson AJ, Abbott JA, Kingston A, et al. Fluoroscopically guided synechiolysis for patients with Asherman's syndrome: menstrual and fertility outcomes. Fertil Steril 2007; 87:405.

Toulis KA, Goulis DG, Farmakiotis D, Georgopoulos NA, Katsikis I, Tarlatzis BC, et al. Adiponectin levels in women with polycystic ovary syndrome: a systematic review and a meta-analysis. *Hum Reprod Update*. May-Jun 2009;15(3):297-307

Van Kruchten PM, Vermelis JM, Herold I, Van Zundert AA (2010). "Hypotonic and isotonic fluid overload as a complication of hysteroscopic procedures: two case reports". *Minerva Anestesiol. 2010 May;76(5):373-7.*

Women with pelvic inflammatory disease: a randomized trial. Obstet Gynecol 2005;106(3):573–80.

Chapter 2

Endoscopy versus IVF: The Way to Go

Atef Darwish

Additional information is available at the end of the chapter

http://dx.doi.org/10.5772/51825

1. Introduction

1.1. Outlines

- Role of endoscopy in infertility. Microsurgical principles, reconstructive concept.
- Can endoscopy omit ART?
- Endoscopy Vs ART
- Advantages of ART over Endoscopy
- Fertility enhancing procedures:
  - Laparoscopic adnexal surgery.
  - Salpingoscopy
  - Hysteroscopy
- Endoscopy prior to ART (routine hysteroscopy, role of laparoscopy (tubes with or withour hydrosalpnix and paratubal cysts, endometrioma).
- Endoscopically-assisted ART.
- Endoscopy for recurrent implantation failure.
- Future of endoscopy in the era of ART and keynote points.

2. Current approaches for infertility management

In modern practice, three schools are competitors for infertility management, namely expectant, endoscopic and assisted reproductive techniques (ART) approaches. There are no RCTs that compare the effectiveness of surgery againsteither IVF or expectant management. The following table demonstrates pros and cons of each approach (1).

2.1. Rationale of expectant therapy

Any treatment should be compared to expectant therapy.

	Expectant treatment	Endoscopic management	ART
Advantages	Safe cheap	-Restores normal anatomy. -Enhances natural pregnancy. -Long-term results	-Time saving Excellent results
Disadvantages	Anxiety Unpredictable outcome	- expensive additional - specialist training -- experience -adverse effects (including ectopic pregnancies), and operative risks. -Unpredictable outcome	-Stress - Expensive - Risky -OHSS -Unpredictable outcome - Per trial result.

Table 1. Lines of infertility management

2.2. Drawbacks of the expectant therapy

- No strict criteria on which to base management decisions.
- Hence, the likelihood of spontaneous pregnancy for each individual couple must be weighed against the potential benefits or risks of interventional treatment.

2.3. Is surgery better than IVF?

Logicstudies: Microsurgical reversal of sterilization is a highly cost-effective strategy when compared with IVF for women aged 40 years and above (2).

Illogic studies: some over enthusiastic studies demonstrated that endoscopy is much better than ART. In a bizarre study, Marana et al. (3) included 43 patientsand subjected them to diagnostic or operative laparoscopy. Nine of themwith submucous-intramural or multiple intramural fibroids underwent miomectomy by minilaparotomy following hysteroscopy and chromopertubation. The mean length of follow- up was 49 months (range: 11 to 118 months). They reported a very high pregnancy rate as 61 became pregnant (40%).

2.4. Advantages of laparoscopy over ART

- Excellent results.
- Long-lasting efficacy.
- Reconstructive concept.
- Physically and psychologically sound patient.

Tubal reconstructive surgery remains an important option for many couples and surgery should be the first line approach for a correct diagnosis and treatment of tubal infertility (4).

2.5. Advantages of endoscopic management over conventional management

- cosmetically most acceptable.
- shorter hospital stay.
- lower incidence of ileus.
- faster recovery.
- less post-operative pain and discomfort, and
- earlier resumption of normal activities and employment.
- reduced contamination of the surgical field with glove powder or lint.
- bleeding is reduced due to tamponade of small vessels by the pneumoperitoneum
- drying of tissues is minimal because surgery occurs in a closed environment
- easy intraoperative access to the pouch of Douglas and the posterior aspects of the genital organ.

2.6. Fertility-preserving reconstructive gynecologic surgery

- **Avoidance of serosal insults:** tissue trauma, ischemia, hemorrhage, infection, foreign-body reaction, and leaving raw surfaces.
- **minimizing tissue trauma:** by using atruamatic techniques, meticulous hemostasis, complete excision of abnormal tissues and precise alignment and approximation of tissue planes .

Evidence of superiority of Laparoscopic reconstructive surgery: one study proved that reconstructive surgery achieves a double pregnancy rate than non-reconstructive surgery (5).

2.7. Is there a role for robotic surgery in improving pregnancy rate?

Among experienced endoscopists, it's well known that it's not the robot that does the surgery, it's the surgeon!

In a retrospective study, both robotically-assisted laparoscopic and standard laparoscopic treatments of endometriosis had excellent outcomes. The robotic technique required significantly longer surgical and anesthesia time, as well as larger trocars (6).

Myth	Facts
Three-D vision	no demonstration that it increasesspeed or safety
The surgeon sees up to 30% more endometriosis.	No RCT
Less recurrence and slowly	No RCT
Rapid recovery and smooth postop course	No RCT
The dexterity (ability to bend at the "wrist") of the robotic instruments makes it possible to perform some surgeries laparoscopically that would otherwise require laparotomy.	this point is debated among experts.

Table 2. Pros and cons of Robotic surgery

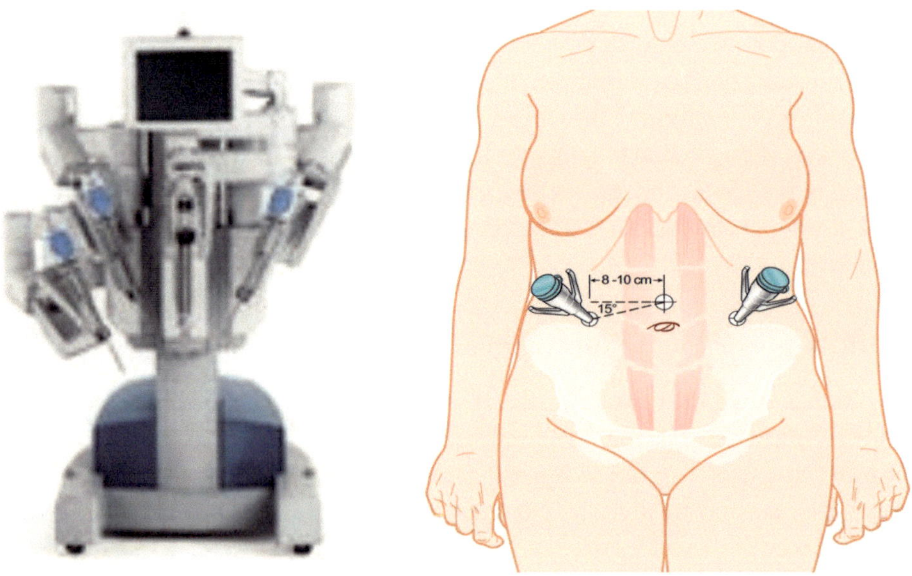

Figure 1. Robotic surgery in Gynecology

2.8. Can IVF replace endoscopy?

Due to advances in the field of IVF/ICSI and stratification of management plans worldwide, the overall pregnancy rate following IVF/ICSI overcame that following endoscopic surgery in many centers. These encouraging results made some authors consider ART superior to surgery and should be offered as a first-line treatment (7).

2.9. Which approach should we use: expectant, endoscopy or ART? (8)

The treatment choice depends upon:

- Severity of the tubal disease.
- Duration of subfertility.
- Maternal age.
- Coexisting infertility factors.

Despite the widespread utilization of assisted reproductive techniques in recent years, hysteroscopic as well as laparoscopic surgery should be firstly offered for patients with adnexal and uterine lesions desiring fertility. Permanent correction of the patient's problem with frequent chances of pregnancy is a definite advantage of endoscopic surgery over assisted reproductive techniques. Reconstructive endoscopic procedures could be performed for fertile women as well e.g. hysteroscopic or laparoscopic myomectomy for abnormal bleeding. The concept of reconstruction following microsurgical principles coupled with refinement of instrumentation and techniques is would improve the results of hysteroscopic and laparoscopic approaches. It is expected to expand to cover many gynecologic aspects in the coming years particularly with the continuous advances in technology of fine endoscopic surgery and the development of more suitable robotic instrumentation.

2.10. Laparoscopy and IVF/ICSI are complementary since a long time (9)

The first in vitro fertilization (IVF) child ensued following the partnership by a scientist with a focused ambition (Nobel laureate Robert Edwards) joining with the gynecologist who introduced laparoscopy to Britain in the late 60's (Patrick Steptoe). Egg retrieval was done laparoscopically. In modern practice, laparoscopic egg retrieval is still required whenever inaccessible ovaries are encountered. A trial of transabdominal sonographic aspiration was recently published with lower success rate of egg retrieval if compared to transvaginal sonographic aspiration (10).

Laparoscopic GIFT: a blastocyst intrafallopian transfer was associated with an intrauterine pregnancy; however, when the indication for blastocyst tubal transfer of an obstructed cervix is associated with a foreshortened cervix requiring cervical cerclage, there can be major health risks for infant and mother (11).

2.11. What's the best approach?

Always try to use the appropriate approach for a suitable couple at the appropriate time. To achieve the best results, try to stratify the lines of management according to pathology putting in mind other circumstances. The following are examples of how to think in each case separately.

3. Pelvic endometriosis: A good example of how to individualize treatment

The optimal management of endometriotic ovarian cysts in infertile patients is less well defined. Recent evidence of reduced responsiveness to gonadotrophins following laparoscopic ovarian cystectomy has challenged the traditional surgical approach to treatment (12). Indeed, it has been suggested that surgery should be undertaken only for the treatment of large endometriomas or pain that is refractory to medical treatment, or to exclude malignancy (13).

Laparoscopic surgery may be of benefit in treating subfertility associated with mild to moderate endometriosis. However, additional studies in this field are needed before definitive conclusions can be drawn (14). Laparoscopic excision of ovarian endometriomas more than 3 cm in diameter may improve fertility. (level II evidence). The effect on fertility of surgical treatment of deeply infiltrating endometriosis is controversial (level II evidence).

3.1. Is there a need to treat endometriosis in patients undergoing IVF?

In a meta-analysis (15)the chance of achieving pregnancy after IVF was significantly lower for patients with endometriosis (odds ratio, 0.56; 95% confidence interval, 0.44-0.70), as compared to those withtubal factor. They also reported decreased fertilization rates, implantation rates and in the number of oocytes retrieved.

3.2. Mild endometriosis Vs severe endometriosis prior to IVF/ICSI

The same study (15) reported that the probability of pregnancy was reduced in women with severe endometriosis as compared to those with mild disease.

Contrarily, a recent retrospective poorly designed study (16) demonstrated that ovarian endometriosis does not reduce IVF outcome compared with tubal factor. Furthermore, laparoscopic removal of endometriomas does not improve IVF results, but may cause a decrease of ovarian responsiveness to gonadotropins. Nevertheless, they included a bizarre group of patients with one or more endometrioma, unilateral or bilateral with a size of6 cm and more importantly symptomatic as well as asymptomatic cases. In addition to being a retrospective analysis, these heterogenous criteria would weaken this study. We believe that stripping off cyst wall of a unilateral endometrioma wouldn't be expected to affect ovarian reserve or ovarian response to gonadotropins.

3.3. Advantages of laparoscopic surgery for endometriosis prior to IVF (ESHRE Recommendations, 2005) (17)

- confirms the diagnosis histologically
- reduces the risk of infection
- improvesaccess to follicles
- Improves ovarian response.

3.4. More advantages include

- Spontaneous pregnancy in mild and moderate disease.
- Elimination of pelvic pain by destruction of the peritneal endometriotic lesions which may be mistaken by OHSS if the patient is subjected to IUI.

3.5. Precautions of laparoscopic surgery prior to IVF/ICSI

- The woman should be counseled regarding the risks of reduced ovarian function after surgery and the loss of the ovary.
- The decision should be reconsidered if she has had previous ovarian surgery.
- RCTs showed that the excision technique is associated with a higher pregnancy rate and a lower rate of recurrence although it may determine severe injury to the ovarian reserve.
- Improvements to this latter aspect may be represented by a combined excision-vaporization technique or by replacing diathermy coagulation with surgical ovarian suture.

4. Role of hysteroscopy prior to assisted reproduction

Failure of IVF treatment can be broadly attributed to embryonic, uterine or transfer factors, but remains unexplained in most cases (18). A number of interventions have been proposed to improve IVF outcome, many of which are not strictly evidence-based and their efficacy in improving pregnancy rates remains controversial (19,20). One of the main causes of failure of implantation after proper embryo transfer is intrauterine pathology. Whether to perform hysteroscopic evaluation of the endometrial cavity prior to IVF/ICSI especially in patients with repeated failures is a controversial issue that is open for criticism and deserves further studies (21).

In a systematic review (Level Ia evidence), 5 reliable studies were included (22). Two RCT showed a statistically significant improvement in the clinical pregnancy rate in the group who had office hysteroscopy (pooled RR = 1.57, 95% CI 1.29–1.92, $P < 0.00001$). The miscarriage rate was not statistically different between the office hysteoscopy and control groups in either study (24% versus 29%, respectively, RR = 0.83, 95% CI 0.56–1.21, $P = 0.33$). Three non-randomized controlled studies suggests that office hysteroscopy improves the pregnancy rate in the subsequent IVF cycle (pooled RR = 2.01, 95% CI 1.60–2.52, $P < 0.00001$). In addition to the well known diagnostic as well as therapeutic advantages of performing hysteroscopy, even if the endometrial cavity was completely free, high pregnancy rate was achieved after diagnostic hysteroscopy since uterine instrumentation during hysteroscopy would inevitably cause a degree of endometrial injury and provokes a posttraumatic reaction that involves release of cytokines and growth factors (23,24), which in turn may influence the likelihood of implantation (25). Commencing IVF treatment soon after hysteroscopy may take advantage of this immunological response (26). Performing diagnostic hysteroscopy before assisted reproductive technologies (ART) may be advisable not only from the clinical but also from the economic point of view (27). Enhanced clinical pregnancy rates would be achieved on adding office hysteroscopy as a complementary step prior to IVFspecially patients with recurrent IVF embryo transfer failures even after normal hysterosalpingography findings. Some abnormal intrauterine findings that would affect the prognosis of IVF/ICSI can be easily diagnosed by hysteroscopy like chronic endometritis, Müllerian anomalies, retained fetal bones, or endocervical ossification. Moreover, contact hysteroscopy may reveal addition valuable findings such as polyposis, strawberry pattern, hypervascularisation, irregular endometrium with endometrial defects, or cystic haemorrhagic lesion which are commonly seen with adenomyosis (28). Future high-quality randomized trials are needed to confirm the favorable effect of standard hysteroscopy in different IVF populations and examine whether newer and less invasive techniques of uterine cavity evaluation such as mini-hysteroscopy (29) or hysterocontrast sonography (30) would have an equally beneficial effect when compared with no intervention before IVF.

With the advent of technical refinements and advancement in hysteroscopic surgery, it is expected that preoperative hysteroscopic evaluation of uteri prior to IVF/ICSI would be widely performed. Unfortunately, many of studies on this topic focus on the central role of hysteroscopic examination of the endometrial cavity in cases with recurrent failures (28,31,32). This concept should be reviewed since office hysteroscopy or minihysteroscopy is a simple outpatient conscious procedure (33-34) that provides excellent information on the implantation site in the endometrial cavity in a very short time. Relying on hysterosalpingography alone may be fallacious in some cases of fine intrauterine adhesions that may be masked by dye especially oily dye. Likewise, transvaginal ultrasonography as well as sonohysterograohy may miss some important fine intrautrerine lesions thatwould simply contribute for failures (3). In one study, hysteroscopy succeeded to diagnose and treat intrauterine lesions in 26% of patients prior to starting trials of assisted reproduction (31). In a big sample sized study (36), intrauterine pathology was diagnosed in about 23% of 2500 cases prior to IVF trial. Another study diagnosed abnormalities in only 11 out of 678 cases. On reevaluation of DVD records of hysteroscopy by an experienced team, the same team reported perfect diagnosis in 77.6% of cases (37).

Following recurrent IVF failure there is some evidence of benefit from hysteroscopy in increasing the chance of pregnancy in the subsequent IVF cycle, both in those with abnormal and normal hysteroscopic findings. Various possible mechanisms have been proposed for this beneficial effect, but more randomized controlled trials are needed before its routine use in the general subfertile population can be recommended (38).

4.1. What is the ideal approach prior to IVF?

In recent years, conflicting opinions on the role of hysteroscopy before any case of IVF/ICSI or after failure once or more times. This conflict is due to different circumstances in different parts of the world regarding:availability of free health insurance for IVF, experienced hysteroscopists, availability of high-resolution 2D ultrasonography with or without SIS, use of office versus conventional hysteroscopes, use of vaginoscopic approach or not and socioeconomic level of the couple. Our opinion is summarized as follows:

- In centers where health insurance is covering the cycles, experienced sonographers performing high-resolution 2D ultrasonography with or without SIS, we believe that they can proceed for IVF without prior hysteroscopy.
- In centers where health insurance is not covering the cycles, experienced sonographers performing high-resolution 2D ultrasonography with or without SIS are not available, we believe that hysteroscopy specially office is very useful in such cases.

- In cases of failed IVF once, hysteroscopy is valuable and recommended.
- In cases with recurrent implantation failure, hysteroscopy is mandatory.

4.2. Office hysteroscopy versus saline-infusion sonography (SIS)

In 1999, we published our first series of SIS for screening in infertile patients utilizing 0.9% saline as an infusion solution and Nelaton catheters for injection (39). We reported satisfactory results. One year later, we published a study (40) on the efficacy of SIS for the detection of endometrial polyps in comparison to the conventional hysteroscopy. These studies compared SIS versus conventional hysteroscopy with excellent results in favor of SIS. Later on, we introduced office hysteroscopy (I use it since 2002 utilizing 2.6 mm telescope). With the advent of vaginoscopic approach, the procedure gained more acceptability among our patients. Now, after these years of experience we changed our mind and strongly say that office hysteroscopy can easily replace indirect diagnostic tools like SIS or 4D ultrasonography. Moreover, more detailed description of the endometrial cavity particularly the blood vessels would be obtained only with office hysteroscopy as we recently published (41).

5. Role of hysteroscopy after embryo transfer

In a study evaluating the incidence of endometrial injury following embryo transfer, office hysteroscopy was performed immediately following embryo transfer and demonstrated marked endocervical and endometrial damage following rigid catheters more than soft catheters (42). Even for cases of early abortion following IVF/ICSI, hysteroscopy was proved to be very valuable. In one study (43), among 84 early abortion patients after IVF-ET, it succeeded to diagnose intrauterine abnormalities in 58 (69.05%) of the patients, including intrauterine adhesion in 32 (32/84, 38.10%), endometrial polyps in 12 (12/84, 14.29%), endometritis in 10 (10/84, 11.90%), submucous leiomyoma in 3 (3/84, 3.57%) and septa in 1 (1/84, 1.19%).

6. Hysteroscopic embryo transfer

As a trial of improving implantation rate following IVF/ICSI, some scattered papers described hysteroscopically-guided embryo transfer. Principally, hysteroscopic approach was selected in difficult cases of embryo transfer (44).

6.1. A new hysteroscopic tubal embryo transfer catheter was developed

Catheterization was performed in 60 patients at hysteroscopic insemination into tube, using 3 French catheters, in which the distal 3,4, and 5 cm tapered to 2 French. Hysteroscopic tubal embryo transfer and conventional IVE-ET were performed in 30 patients with normal tubes, who failed to achieve pregnancy after 2 IVF-ET trials. The success rate of complete insertion with the catheter tapering at the distal 3 cm was significantly higher than that at the distal 5 cm. Since we obtained the highest success rate of insertion with the catheter tapering at the distal 3 cm, we selected this catheter for the h-TEST. The rate of pregnancy in h-TEST was significantly higher than that in conventional ET (45).

6.2. Hysteroscopic Endometrial Embryo Delivery (HEED) (46)

It refers to visually confirmed placement of the embryo(s) at a specific area on the surface of the uterus. It is done in an office setting, using a special fiberoptic scope and camera plus special tubing, and it takes approximately two minutes to perform. It uses nitrogen gas to avoid deleterious effect of CO2 gas o n the embryos. HEED can also be used for earlier (day 2 or 3) embryos as well as the more advanced embryos. This is especially advantageous in situations where the numbers of embryos are limited, or embryo quality is of concern. It is particularly useful in patients with advanced reproductive age, or when egg production is low, or in patients with poor sperm parameters. Patients will actually see the process on video monitor. The entry into the uterus is not always easy, as the non-stirrable tip of the catheter must usually go through different curvatures in the cervical canal and the uterine cavity while minimizing injury to the lining of the uterus, before it reaches the final destination. The flexible hysteroscope has a stirrable tip, helping guide the endoscope in a gas expanded uterine cavity. The slightly expanded uterine cavity also helps avoid contact between the hysteroscope and uterine surface. The final destination of the tip of the catheter is visually confirmed. This more precise placement and lower volume of transfer fluid may help reduce incidence of ectopic pregnancies even further. It may also reduce chances placenta previa, where the after birth is lying over the uterine opening. Presence of uterine contraction at the time of transfer that are otherwise not noticeable by using the "Blind" embryo transfer technique, can be visually confirmed and embryo transfer deferred. Precise and visually confirmed placement, may reduce percentage of multiple pregnancies, by reducing number of embryos transferred because of the less uncertainty of the placement of embryos with the "Blind" technique. Nevertheless, since the embryo(s) are laid on top of the uterine surface, due to inherent uterine contractions over the next few days after the embryo delivery and prior to their natural implantation in the uterine cavity, the embryo(s) may be expelled either into the fallopian tube (causing ectopic pregnancy) or out of the uterus, as they do with the current "blind" embryo transfer technique.

6.3. Subendometrial embryo delivery (SEED) (47)

Patients will actually see the process on video monitor. It will reduce the chances that the embryo will fall out of the uterus, or that it will fall into the fallopian tube causing tubal pregnancy. Post embryo implantation, the woman does NOT need to stay in bed for 2 days.

The main disadvantage includes a possible scratching of the lining of the uterus so that pregnancy may not ensue. Candidates include any patient undergoing IVF, specially patients with previously failed standard embryo transfers, patients with ectopic pregnancies and tubal disease.

It is done in an office setting using a special fiberoptic scope and camera plus a special tubing with a needlepoint, and it takes approximately two minutes to perform. It utilizes flexible hysteroscope and an inert gas (nitrous gas) to avoid the deleterious effect of CO2 gas on the embryos.

6.4. Hysteroscopic cervical canal refashioning prior to difficult embryo transfer (48)

In some cases, access to the endometrial cavity is extremely difficult or even impossible. In some scarce studies. Sonographically-guided fine needle transmyometrial embryo transfer was tried but this technique is not universally accepted. An attractive recent hysteroscopic approach was described. The procedure is performed under general anesthesia. Patients are taken into the theater with a full bladder in case ultrasound guidance is required to access the uterine cavity. A Versapoint electrode (twizzle electrode) with a 1.9 mm Versascope (Gynecare division, Johnson and Johnson) is used for the procedure. The Versapoint electrode works on bipolar energy, so saline is used as the distension media. Versascope sheath has a small diameter (3.5 mm) and it can be inserted into the cervical canal without prior dilatation or with minimal dilatation. In two patients the canal is extremely tortuous and fibrotic and it is not possible to negotiate with the delicate Versascope. Cervical dilatation is achieved under ultrasound guidance in these women and the Versapoint twizzle electrode is introduced through the operating channel of an operating hysteroscope (Olympus).

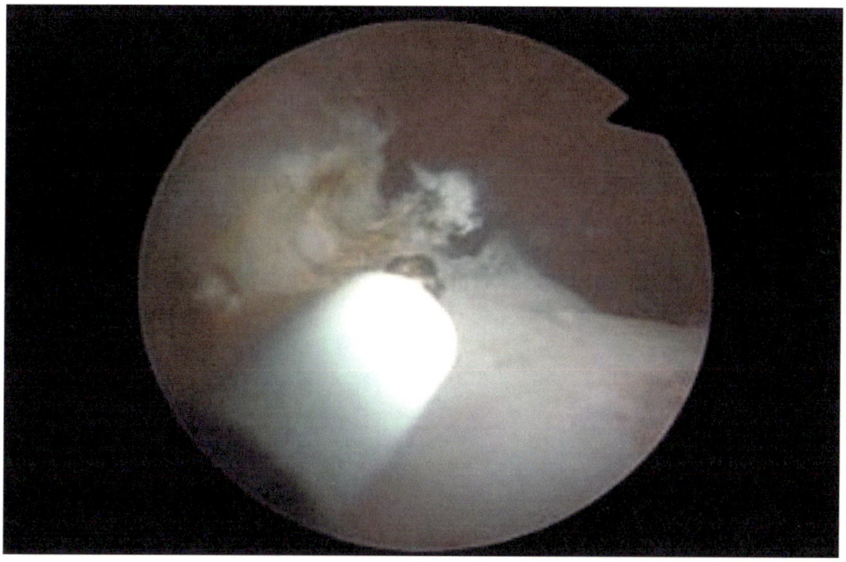

Figure 2. Hysteroscopic cervical canal refashoning

For women with a false passage and acute angulation of the uterus, the tissue between the actual cervical canal and false passage is cut thus leaving a clean path which could be negotiated with an ET catheter. For the problem of a severely fibrotic OS, 1 or 2 linear releasing incisions are made with the Versapoint electrode, extending from the posterior aspect of the internal OS towards the external OS for approximately 1 cm. In patients who had a tortuous cervical canal, several projecting ridges are seen arising from the anterior, posterior and/or lateral walls of the cervical canal. The hysteroscope is introduced into the uterine cavity and then withdrawn towards the external OS. As the hysteroscope is moved outwards the cervical canal projections distorting linearity of the canal are visualized. Linear releasing incisions of approximately a centimeter are made into these projections and a straightening of the canal is achieved. Subsequent to the procedure, dilatation is done to further stretch the incised fibrous tissue, and it is now possible to dilate the cervix up to size 10/12 Hegar in even the most resistant cervix.

6.5. Hysteroscopic site-specific endometrial injury (49)

A site-specific hysteroscopic biopsy-induced injury of the endometrium during the controlled ovarian hyperstimulation cycle has been shown to improve subsequent embryo implantation in patients with repeated implantation failure. The procedure starts with performing panoramic hysteroscopy. A flexible claw forceps is introduced through a 2.2 mm working channel which is used to generate a local injury on the posterior endometrium at midline 10-15 mm from the fundus on D4 to D7 of the stimulation cycle. The depth and width of the injured site is 2 × 2 mm (i.e. a bite of the claw forceps). No antibiotic or hemostatic drug is administered after the procedure.

Endometrial injury may have a beneficial role in implantation and improve the pregnancy rate. However, there are still many unanswered question including patients selection, timing, technique and number of endometrial biopsies needed (50).

7. Role of endoscopy in cases of hydrosalpnix

- Tubal pathology, particularly hydrosalpinx, is associated with a low embryo implantation rate in IVF as well as an increased risk for early pregnancy loss.
- The role of surgery for tubal disease to improve IVF outcomes, in the absence of hydrosalpinx, requires further evaluation.

In recent years, considerable attention has been given to the possible impact of the presence of hydrosalpinx on implantation and ongoing pregnancy rates following IVF/ICSI (51,52). The mechanism of disruption remains uncertain. However, proposed mechanisms may be attributed to alteration in endometrial receptivity ordirect embryo toxic effect (53). Furthermore, hydrosalpnix is liable be unintentionally punctured at the time of egg retrieval or it may disturb the access to the ovary if it is too big. A systematic review of three RCTs (54) showed that tubal surgery such as laparoscopic salpingectomy significantly increased live birth rate (OR 2.13; 95% CI 1.24 to 3.65) and pregnancy rate (OR 1.75; 95% CI 1.07 to 2.86) in women with hydrosalpinges before IVF when compared with no treatment. There are no significant differences in the odds of ectopicpregnancy (OR 0.42; 95% CI 0.08 to 2.14), miscarriage (OR 0.49; 95% CI 0.16 to 1.52), treatment complication (OR 5.80; 95% CI 0.35 to 96.79) or implantation (OR 1.34; 95% CI 0.87to 2.05). Since hydrosalpinx reduces IVF pregnancy rates (14,55), it is therefore suggested that women with hydrosalpinges should be offered diagnostic/operative laparoscopy and a trial of salpingoneostomy. If failed or inaccessable, salpingectomy could be offered prior to IVF/ICSI to improve the chance of a live birth. Sometimes, laparoscopic access to the isthmic part of the tube is not feasible even in experienced hands particularly in patients with history of repeated laparotomies, intestinal reanastomosis, or kidney transplantation. This situation may pave the way to hysteroscopic occlusion of the fallopian tubes based on the reported success in hysteroscopic tubal cannulation and sterilization techniques. The effectiveness of draining of hydrosalpinges or performing salpingostomy on improving live birth rate prior to IVF/ICSI needs further evaluation.

7.1. Methods of endoscopic proximal occlusion of functionless and harmful hysrosalpnix

1. **Laparoscopic:** this can be easily performed using a bipolar grasping forceps or monopolar grasping forceps. In either approach, take care to apply a little traction on the tube medially to avoid scattered secondary coagulation towards the lateral pelvic wall particularly when utilizing monopolar diathermy. By this way, the ureter would be perfectly secured. Some center using clips.
2. **Hysteroscopic:** this approach can be performed whenever laparoscopic approach is impossible or dangerous like cases with history of extensive abdominal surgery like resection anastomosis of the intestine or previous colonic surgery, or patients with a history of extensive or recurrent surgery for pelvic endometriosis. Practically, endoscopists may face some cases without feasibility to perform laparoscopy from the start. These cases deserve searching for an alternative approaches. Hysteroscopy comes as an attractive valuable alternative. Some studies used Essure devices to hysteroscopically occlude the proximal part of the fallopian tube. They reported some case reports of successful pregnancy. Nevertheless, we believe that leaving a foreign body in-utero would lead to decreasing implantation rate. Herein, I'll discuss in details our previous unique study on hysteroscopic tubal occlusion in cases with hydrosalpnix (56). The in-vitro safety phase of this study is done on fresh uterine specimens removed by abdominal or vaginal hysterectomy. In this phase the study, fresh hysterectomy specimens are placed on the return electrode of diathermy, then the corneal ends of both tubes are coagulated simulating the same manner as in the clinical phase. Temperature study is done using digital thermometer over the uterine serosa at site of the coagulation. Histopathologic sections are made to assess tissue effects and depth of penetration using Nitro Blue Tetrazolium (NBT) to evaluate the extent of coagulation on the tubal uterine junction. Computerized image analyzer (Leica Q 500 MB Computerized Image Analyzer) is used to measure the depth of diathermy damage to the surrounding myometrium. The clinical phase of this study is conducted at the out-patient Infertility clinic of Women Health hospital, Assiut University, from April 2004 to October 2006 and included 27 patients with definite uni- or bilateral laparoscopically-proved functionless hydrosalpinges scheduled for IVF/ICSI. All patients gave a written consent and the study is approved by the institutional ethics committee. They were randomly divided into 2 groups. Randomization is done using simple computer generated randomization tables method. Group A comprised 14 patients who were randomly allocated for laparoscopic occlusion. Laparoscopy is performed under general endotracheal anesthesia using a standard double puncture technique. Once the

peritoneal cavity is entered, a panoramic evaluation of the pelvis is done. If the pelvis looks frozen or if the access to the fallopian tubes is impossible, the patient is considered failed laparoscopic approach. Those cases are subsequently treated by open laparotomic or hysteroscopic approach but the results of these procedures are not included in this study. If the procedure seems feasible, a third auxillary puncture is done. Utilizing a bipolar forceps, the isthmic part of the fallopian tube is coagulated and incised to ensure complete tubal occlusion as a case of tubal sterilization. The procedure is completed after securing hemostasis. The patient is discharged after 3-4 hours under antibiotic prophylaxis. Group B included 13 patients scheduled for hysteroscopic approach. The cervix is primed in all cases using 200 Mg misoprostol 8 hours prior to the procedure as previously described (57). The procedure is done immediately postmenstrual without specific preparation. Local paracervical anesthesia is selected in 5 cases while spinal anesthesia in 6 cases, and general anesthesia in 2 cases. Selection of the anesthestic technique is chosen according to patient preference after proper explanation by the anesthiologist. The cervix is gently dilated till Hegar's 10 which is followed by insertion of a rotatory continuous flow monopolar resectoscope. Once the peritubal pulge (the proximal part of the intramural segment of the tubeis clearly seen, a roller ball electrode of 3 mm size is bluged inside it and activated at 50 watts for about 8 seconds. A thorough comment on the fundus and the rest of the endometrial cavity is reported. The patients are discharged immediately if the procedure is done under local paracervical anesthesia, while the remaining cases are discharged few hours later. In both groups, the procedure is preceded and done under prophylactic broad spectrum antibiotic coverage to guard against any risk of flaring up of infection of the functionless hydrosalpnix. In both groups, patients are instructed to come back the next cycle postmenstually where hysterosalpingography (HSG) is done for most cases especially those with unilateral functionless hydrosalpnix. If the patient refused and has bilateral hydrosalpnix, sonohysterography (SHG) is done utilizing a simplified technique as previously described (39). Tubal occlusion of the affected side is confirmed if marked resistance is encountered on repeated injection of saline without evidence of intraperitoneal leakage from the occluded side which is the main outcome measure. Second-look office hysteroscopy is done for patients in group B whenever possible. The in-vitro safety phase resulted in bilateral complete coagulation of the proximal part of the tubes with secondary coagulation shown of up to 3 mm as shown in the histopathologic sections. When the power of coagulation is 50-60 W and operating time not prolonged more than 20 seconds , the thermal damage covered corneal end as complete coagulation in addition to2mm -3 mm secondary coagulation of the adjacent cornualendo- myometrium. Serosal temperature is not exceeding 41.9 Cº (range 39 Cº - 41.9 Cº) at any time during the procedure. No full thickness injuries are demonstrated either histologically or suggested by the temperature studies. Hysteroscopic access is achieved in 12 (85.7%)and occlusion is achieved in 9 (64.2%) cases. If the peritubal pulge is not clearly visible, the case is considered as failed access to the proper site of occlusion. In group B, diagnostic hysteroscopy showed fine marginal adhesions in 2 cases (15%) and a small polyp in one case (7.7%). Hysteroscopic tubal occlusion showed shorter operative time (9 ±2.76 min vs. 23.6 ±4.75 min, p= 0.0001) and hospital stay as well (2 ±1.84 hours vs. 5 ±1.13 hours, p= 0.0001). No case of intraoperative complication in either group is reported. There is no case of exaggerated postoperative pelvic pain or fever in either group. HSG or SHG demonstrated complete tubal occlusion of the affected side in all cases in both groups). Second-look office hysteroscopy is done in 8 cases of group B which revealed no significant corneal lesions at the site of hysteroscopic occlusion. Pregnancy is achieved in 4 (28.5%) and 4(30.7%) cases in both groups respectively following IVF/ICSI without any significant difference between both groups.

7.2. Comments on hysteroscopic tubal occlusion in hydrosalpnix

Hysteroscopic tubal occlusion of functionless hydrosdalpngies is a unioque one. It demonstrates a valuable role of hysteroscopic approach that can be performed in difficult cases with poor access to the isthmic part of the tubes via laparoscopy even with experienced hands. The idea is attractive but further large-sample sized studies are required to define the exact role of this approach.

One of the interesting additive items of this paper to the literature is the term "functionless" hydrosalpnix. The proposed definition is very crucial to stratify cases suitable for microsurgical salpingoneotomy and those cases suitable for occlusive procedures. By this way, the place of reconstructive surgery is still preserved in modern practice even in the era of IVF/ICSI. Ethically, every effort should be exerted to restore normal anatomy whenever possible. This concept is of utmost importance particularly for the developing countries with limited resources where no national programs to support assisted reproductive techniques. Microsurgery to correct localized damage has the advantage of long-standing restoration of fertility. A simple prognostic classification is lacking. The severity of the tubal damage and the health of the mucosa is key in determining outcome. Proper selection of the tube for either line of management requires expert knowledge with the principles of salpingoscopy. Salpingoscopy during laparoscopy yields the best prognosis in patients with hydrosalpinx. Performing salpingoscopy with laparoscopy could significantly increase accuracy in predicting short-term fertility outcome. Whenever the mucosa is unhealthy, surgery is not justified; early referral for IVF is indicated.

Hysteroscopic tubal occlusion of proximal part of the hydrosalpnix is feasible and promising as a safe, effective, fast, and easy approach. It can be done as an out-patient procedure under local paracervical block. It has the advantage of adding valuable evaluation of the endometrial cavity prior to IVF/ICSI. Further large sample-sized studies are required specially those utilizing bipolar resectoscope. The impact of hysteroscopic tubal occlusion on subsequent implantation and pregnancy rates needs to be addressed in another larger study. Since it is a preliminary study, the current role of hysteroscopic occlusion should be limited to cases of failed laparoscopic approach. Further studies are required before moving hysteroscopic occlusion to replace laparoscopic occlusion prior to IVF/ICSI.

7.3. A suggested flowchart for management of functionless hydrosalpnix prior to IVF/ICSI

Laparoscopic tubal surgery: tubal factors include proximal tubal occlusion, distal tubal phimosis or occlusion or peritubal adhesions. Endoscopy (whether laparoscopy or hysteroscopy) play a central role in the management of tubal disease.

- Tubal pathology, particularly hydrosalpinx, is associated with a low embryo implantation rate in IVF as well as an increased risk for early pregnancy loss.
- The role of surgery for tubal disease to improve IVF outcomes, in the absence of hydrosalpinx, requires further evaluation.

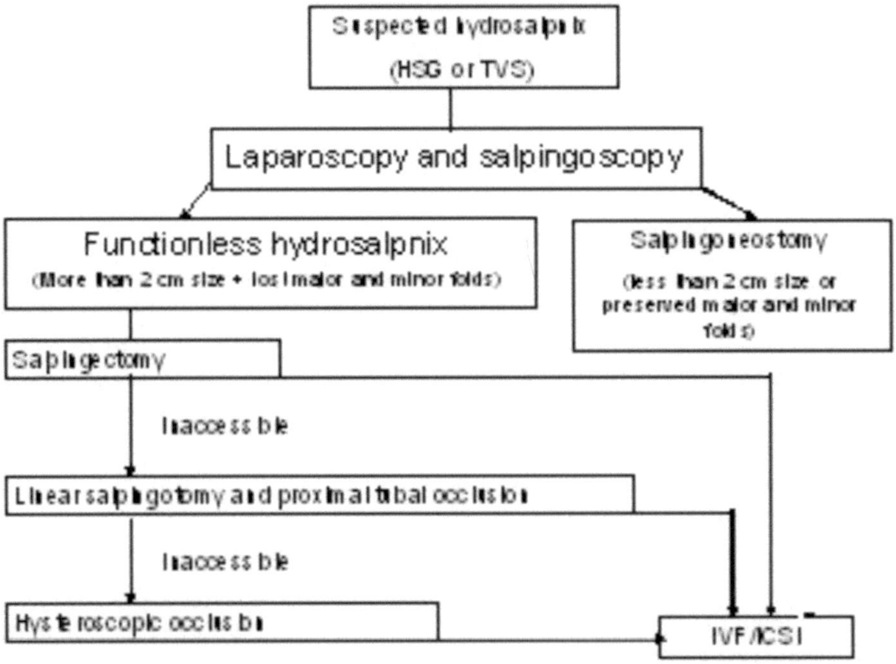

Figure 3. **HSG:** Hysterosalpingography. **TVS:** Transvaginal ultrasonography.

7.4. Laparoscopic management of distal tubal disease

Distal tubal occlusion may be due to hydrosalpnix, pyosalpnix or peritubal adhesions. Obstruction of the distal fallopian tube is one of the most common causes of female infertility (58). In cases of pyosalpnix, just tubal opening, drainage of pus and proper peritoneal toilet are sufficient. Don't forget to take a tubal wall biopsy. Don't proceed for tubal occlusion at the same setting for fear of disseminating infection and the possibility of tubal bilharziasis with reported cases of spontaneous pregnancy after proper treatment. Nowadays, it is conceived that the presence of hydrosalpinx is associated with a compromised outcome for IVF/ ICSI. Hydrosalpinx is associated with lower implantation and fecundibility rates even if the contralateral tube is sound which may be attributed to alteration in endometrial receptivity

(59) or direct embryo toxic effect. Furthermore, it is liable to be unintentionally punctured at the time of egg retrieval or it may disturb access to the ovary if it is too big. In a meta-analysis, it has been demonstrated that there is a reduction by half in the probability of achieving a pregnancy in the presence of hydrosalpinx, and an almost doubled rate of spontaneous abortion (60). In an animal study, hydrosalpinx fluid is shown to contain toxins that are potentially teratogenic (61). Proposed mechanisms of impaired implantation rate due to hydrosalpinges are well addressed in the literature (62). Selected patients with unilateral hydrosalpinges and a patent contralateral Fallopian tube may exhibit increased cycle fecundity after salpingectomy or proximal tubal occlusion of the affected tube, and may conceive without the need for IVF. In a retrospective case-control study, bilateral salpingectomy due to hydrosalpinges restored a normal delivery as well as implantation rate after IVF treatment compared to controls (63). Randomized controlled trials recommended performing laparoscopic salpingectomy prior to IVF, especially inpatients with ultrasound-visible hydrosalpinges (64). In a Cochrane review (65), it is concluded that further randomized trials are required to assess other surgical treatments for hydrosalpinx, such as salpingostomy, tubal occlusion or needle drainage of a hydrosalpinx at oocyte retrieval. Functionless hydrosalpinx can be defined as a large blocked tube with lost major and minor folds, as seen at salpingoscopy after laparoscopic salpingoneostomy.

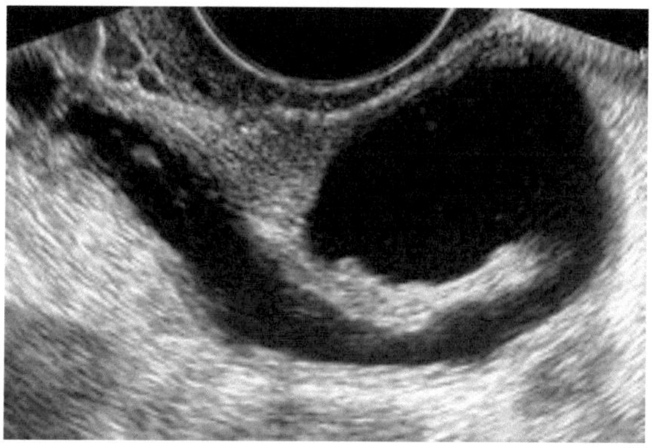

Figure 4. Sonographic appearance of a typical hydrosalpnix.

On sonography, the dilated fallopian tube presents as a thin- or thick-walled tubular fluid-filled structure that may be elongated or folded (figure). Longitudinal folds that are present in a normal fallopian tube may become thickened in the presence of a hydrosalpinx. The dilated fallopian tube may or may not show longitudinal folds. These longitudinal folds are pathognomonic of a hydrosalpinx . If the elongated nature of these folds is not noted, they may be mistaken for mural nodules of an ovarian cystic mass. Identification of a separate ovary helps distinguish a hydrosalpinx from a cystic ovarian mass, an important distinction because malignancy is rare with an extraovarian cystic adnexal mass. A significantly scarred hydrosalpinx may present as a multilocular cystic mass with multiple septa creating multiple compartments. These septa are generally incomplete, and the compartments can be connected. However, with more pronounced scarring, differentiation from an ovarian mass may not be possible (66). Potential pitfalls in the diagnosis of hydrosalpinx include paratubal, paraovarian, or perineural cysts. In some cases, CT or MRI may be helpful to differentiate these conditions from a hydrosalpinx (67).

7.5. Technical tricks of laparoscopic management of hydrosalpnix

a. **Salpingoneostomy:** One of the keys of success is to evaluate the tube externally and internally. If peritubal adhesions exist, microsurgical adhesiolysis should be performed at first. Be sure that the tube is freely mobile. Imagine the site of the new ostium before dealing with the hydroslpnix. It should be directed towards the pouch of Douglas to help ovum pick-up. Start by salpingoneostomy using a fine monopolar or bipolar needle. The finest the needle, the better ostium. Incise the distended distal part of the tube " + shaped" (cruciate incision). Then, evaluate the tubal mucosa using a salpingoscopy. Practically, use the diagnostic hysteroscopy which consists of a 4 mm telescope and a 5 mm outer sheath. Connect it to a normal IV infusion set and use saline as an irrigating fluid. Grasp the new ostium with an atruamatic grasping forceps and insert the hysteroscope with comment on the major and minor folds till reaching the narrowest part of the tube. If major and minor folds are lost this means that the prognosis is poor even after proper refashioning. The next step is to grasp the tubal lumen with atruamatic forcpes and to evert it outside. Lastly, fix the edges of the new ostium either with monopolar spray coagulation just distal to the incised parts to evert them or with the aid of fine sutures.

b. **Salpingectomy:** This procedure is indicated if a pathologic unilateral huge hydrosalpnix is present to enhance spontaneous pregnancy or bilateral big hydrosalpnix before IVF/ICSI. It is performed in the same manner as mentioned in the section of EP.

c. **Tubal occlusion:** Once the peritoneal cavity is entered, a panoramic evaluation of the pelvis is performed. If the pelvis looked frozen or if access to the fallopian tubes is impossible, the patient is considered a failed laparoscopic approach. Those cases are subsequently treated by open laparotomic or hysteroscopic approach. If the procedure seems feasible, a third auxiliary puncture is carried out. Utilizing a bipolar forceps, the isthmic part of the fallopian tube is coagulated and incised to ensure complete tubal occlusion, as a case of tubal sterilization. The procedure is completed after securing hemostasis. The patient is discharged after 3-4 h under antibiotic prophylaxis. Laparoscopic salpingectomy or bipolar proximal tubal occlusion yielded statistically similar responses to controlled ovarian hyperstimulation and IVF-ET cycle outcome. Proximal occlusion might be preferable in patients who present with dense pelvic adhesions and easy access only to the proximal fallopian tube (68). Occlusion is considered a minimally invasive procedure, requires less experience, feasible in most cases, and has fewer burdens on the psychological status of those infertile women. Hysteroscopic approach is recently described by our team at Assiut University Institution (69). The cervix is primed in all cases using misoprostol (200 μg) 8 h prior to the procedure. The procedure is carried out immediately postmenstrual without specific preparation. Local paracervical, spinal or general anesthesia could be used. Selection of the anaesthetic technique is chosen according to patient preference after proper explanation by the anaesthesiologist. The cervix is gently dilated with Hegar 10 and a rotatory continuous flow monopolar resectoscope is inserted. Once the peritubal bulge (the proximal part of the intramural segment of the tubeis clearly seen, a roller ball electrode (size: 3 mm) is introduced inside it and activated at 50 Watts for about 8 seconds. A thorough comment on the fundus and the rest of the endometrial cavity should be reported. The patients are usually discharged immediately if the procedure is carried out under local paracervical anesthesia, while the remaining cases are discharged a few hours later.

8. Proximal tubal occlusion

Usually diagnosed by HSG and confirmed by laparoscopic chromopertubation test. The most important job of the endoscopist is to find out contraindications for hysteroscopic tubal cannulation procedure which include:

- florid infection
- genital tuberculosis
- obliterative fibrosis and long tubal obliterations that are difficult to bypass with the catheter.
- severe tubal damage.
- previously performed tubal surgery.
- salpingitis isthmica nodosa.
- isthmic occlusion with club-changed terminal, ampullar or fimbrial occlusion, and tubal fibrosis
- coaxial TO: combined distal and proximal tubal occlusion.

Don't try to cannulate the tube in such cases as failure would be expected and you would be disappointed. In cases with isolated tubal occlusion, cannulation would be successful.

9. The following is our protocol for tubal disease management

- Pathologic PTO: IVF
- Isolated PTO: TC
- Midsegment O: IVF
- Small hydrosalpnix+ normal salpingoscope:OL
- Functionless hydrosalpnix: PTO then IVF
- Combined PTO and DTO: IVF
- Peritubal adhesions: OL Vs IVF

10. Endoscopic uterine surgery

10.1. Endoscopic myomectomy prior to IVF/ICSI

The impact of uterine myoma on the outcome of IVF/ICSI is a very controversial topic. Many centers are overdoing myomectomy for nearly all myomata regardless size and site considerations. Contrary, other investigators have shown that fibroids don't exert a deleterious effect. Nevertheless, many studies have provided evidence that uterine myomas have a significant effect on IVF outcomes and there is a large body of evidence that treatment of uterine myomas increases fertility and pregnancy rates, and decreases the rate of pregnancy loss (70). There is no doubt that any cavity-distorting myoma should be removed whether completely submucous or interstitial myoma with submucous encroachment. This highlights the central role of prior hysteroscopy as well as saline infusion solonhysterography (SIS) as previously described (39). Not only does sub mucous myoma cause mechanicl interference with implantation, but it also alters endometrial receptivity (71)

Controversy exists for interstitial and subserous myomata. The evidence supports treatment of all very large myomas (>7 cm) (70). Subserosal myomas that are smaller than 7 cm in size and intramural myomas of less than 4–5 cm in diameter appear to have little effect on IVF outcomes. Larger intramural and subserosal myomas present a clinical dilemma and more studies are needed to clarify a definitive plan for management (70). In a prospective controlled study, the distance between the intramural myomas and the endometrial lining did not appear to affect the IVF outcome. An insignificant tendency towards improvement of IVF outcome is found in myomas at more than 5 mm from endometrial lining (72).

In a recent review of literature (73) on myoma and assisted reproduction technology and spontaneous conception, hysteroscopic sub-mucous myoma resection is found to increase pregnancy rates. Intramural fibroids appear to decrease fertility, but the myomectomy does not improve assisted reproduction technology and spontaneous fertility. More high-quality studies are needed to conclude toward the value of myomectomy for intramural fibroids. Subserosal fibroids do not affect fertility outcomes, and removal does not confer benefit.

11. Keynote points

11.1. Tubal infertility

Endoscopy and ART arenot competitors but complementary.

First trial is the best trial for tubal surgery.

Performing laparoscopic surgery Forendometriosis prior to IVF isveryvaluable in manycases.

There is NO adequate trialscomparing pregnancy rates with tubal surgeryversus IVF.

Per cycle pregnancy rate of IVF: higher

Tubal anastomosis for reversal ofsterilization has significantly higher cummulative pregnancy rate than IVF and ismore cost effective even above 40 years.

Factors affecting counseling for tubal surgery or IVF:

- Age of the woman.
- Ovarian reserve.
- Number and quality of sperms/ejaculate.

- Number of children desired.
- Site and extent of tubal disease.
- The presence of other infertility factors.
- The risk of ectopic pregnancy.
- The experience of the surgeon.
- The success rate of IVF program.
- The patient preference.

11.2. Uterine myoma and infertility

Uterine myoma may affect fertility according to its size, site and associated pathology. Endoscopic approach has a definite role in its management. HM is the gold standard line of management of submucous myoma of suitable size. LM doesn't seem to be superior to conventional open myomectomy regarding fertility and is characterized by both short and long term drawbacks. Uterine myomata would affect IVF/ICSI outcome whenever disturbing the endometrial cavity or large sized. The impact of other types of myomata on IVF/ICSI deserves further studies. Hysteroscopic myomectomy is indicated for intracavitary myomas and submucous myomas having at least 50% of their volume within the uterine cavity. The management of the subfertile women with small intramural fibroids (<5 cm) is still a subject of debate (75,76).

Author details

Atef Darwish
Obstetrics and Gynecology, Assiut University, Assiut, Egypt

12. References

[1] Pandian Z, Akande VA, Harrild K, Bhattacharya S. Surgery for tubal infertility. Cochrane Database Syst Rev 2008; Issue 3. Art. No.: CD006415.

[2] Petrucco OM, Silber SJ, Chamberlain SL, Warnes GM, Davies M. Live birth following day surgery reversal of female sterilisation in women older than 40 years: a realistic option in Australia? Med J Aust 2007; 187:271-3.

[3] Marana R, Ferrari S, Merola A, Astorri AL, Pompa G, Milardi D, Giampietro A, Lecca A, Marana E. Role of a mini-invasive approach in the diagnosis and treatment of tubo-peritoneal infertility as an alternative to IVF . Minerva Ginecol. 2011 Feb;63(1):1-10.

[4] Muzii L, Sereni MI, Battista C, Zullo MA, Tambone V, Angioli R Tubo-peritoneal factor of infertility: diagnosis and treatment. Clin Ter. 2010;161(1):77-85.

[5] Bateman BG, Nunley WC Jr, Kitchin JD 3rd. Surgical management of distal tubal obstruction--are we making progress? Fertil Steril. 1987 Oct;48(4):523-42

[6] Nezhat C, Lewis M, Kotikela S, Veeraswamy A, Saadat L, Hajhosseini B, NezhatC. Robotic versus standard laparoscopy for the treatment of endometriosis.Fertil Steril. 2010 Dec;94(7):2758-60.

[7] Feinberg EC, Levens ED, DeCherney AH. Fertil Steril. Infertility surgery is dead: only the obituary remains? 2008 Jan;89(1):232-6.
[8] ASRM Practice Committee. The role of tubal reconstructive surgery in the era of assisted reproductive technologies. Fertil Steril 2008; S250–S253.
[9] Yovich JL. A clinician's personal view of assisted reproductive technology over 35 years. Reprod Biol. 2011 Dec;11 Suppl 3:31-42.
[10] Barton SE, Politch JA, Benson CB, Ginsburg ES, GargiuloAR Transabdominal follicular aspiration for oocyte retrieval in patients with ovaries inaccessible by transvaginal ultrasound. Fertil Steril. 2011 Apr;95(5):1773-6.
[11] Murray A, Hutton J.Successful tubal blastocyst transfer after laparoscopic cervical cerclage: cesarean delivery of a live very low-birth-weight infant and later hysterectomy for uterine rupture. Fertil Steril. 2011 Oct;96(4):895-7. Epub 2011 Jul 30.
[12] Somigliana E, Vercellini P, Vigano P, Ragni G, Crosignani PG. Should endometriomas be treated before IVF-ICSI cycles? Hum Reprod Update 2006;12:57-64
[13] Garcia-Velasco JA, Somigliana E. Management of endometriomas in women requiring IVF: to touch or not to touch. Hum Reprod 2009;24:496-501.).
[14] Jacobsonet al., 2010 Cochrane
[15] Barnhart K, Dunsmoor-Su R, Coutifaris C. Effect of endometriosis on in vitro fertilization. Fertil Steril. 2002 Jun;77(6):1148-55.
[16] Francesca Bongioanni,[1] Alberto Revelli,[2] Gianluca Gennarelli,[2] Daniela Guidetti,[1] Luisa Delle Delle Piane,[2] and Jan HolteOvarian endometriomas and IVF: a retrospective case-control study. prod Biol Endocrinol. 2011; 9: 81.
[17] ESHRE guidelines for the diagnosis and treatment of endometriosis. 2005 www.endometriosis.org
[18] Hamou J: Electroresection of fibroids. In Endoscopic Surgery for Gynaecologists. Ed by Sutton C and Diamond M. London. Sauhders Co LTD, 1993, Ch41.
[19] Margalioth EJ, Ben Chetrit A, Gal M, Eldar Geva T. Investigation and treatment of repeated implantation failure following IVF-ET. Human Reproduction 2006;21, 3036–3043.
[20] Urman B, Yakin K, Balaban B. Recurrent implantation failure in assisted reproduction: how to counsel and manage. A. General considerations and treatment options that may benefit the couple. Reproductive BioMedicine Online 2005; 11, 371–381.
[21] De Sutter P. Rational diagnosis and treatment in infertility. Best Practice and Research in Clinical Obstetrics and Gynaecology 2006; 20, 647–664.
[22] Tarek El-Toukhy, Sesh Kamal Sunkara, Arri Coomarasamy, Jan Grace, Yakoub Khalaf. Outpatient hysteroscopy and subsequent IVF cycle outcome: a systematic review and meta-analysis. Reprod Biomed Online. 2008;16 (5):712-9.
[23] Sharkey A. Cytokines and implantation. Reviews of Reproduction 1998; 3, 52–61.
[24] Basak S, Dubanchet S, Zourbas S. Expression of proinflammatory cytokines in mouse blastocysts during implantation: modulation by steroids hormones. American Journal of Reproductive Immunology2002;47, 2–11.

[25] Raziel A, Schachter M, Strassburger D. Favourable influence of local injury to the endometrium in intracytoplasmic sperm injection patients with high-order implantation failure. Fertility and Sterility 2007; 87, 198–201.
[26] Lea RG, Sandra O. Immunoendocrine aspects of endometrial function and implantation. Reproduction 2007; 134, 389–404.
[27] La Sala, G.B., Montanari, R., Dessanti, L, Cigarini C, Sartori F. The role of diagnostic hysteroscopy and endometrial biopsy in Assisted Reproductive Technologies. Fertil. Steril. 1998; 70, 378–380.
[28] Rama Raju GA, Shashi Kumari G, Krishna KM, Prakash GJ, Madan K. Assessment of uterine cavity by hysteroscopy in assisted reproduction programme and its influence on pregnancy outcome. Arch Gynecol Obstet. 2006;274(3):160-4.
[29] De Placido G, Clarizia R, Cadente C. Compliance and diagnostic efficacy of mini-hysteroscopy versus traditional hysteroscopy in infertility investigation. European Journal of Obstetrics and Gynecology and Reproductive Biology 2007; 135, 83–87.
[30] Tur-Kaspa I, Gal M, Hartman M. A prospective evaluation of uterine abnormalities by saline infusion sonohysterography in 1,009 women with infertility or abnormal uterine bleeding. Fertil Steril 2006; 86, 1731–1735.
[31] Oliveira FG, Abdelmassih VG, Diamond MP, Dozortsev D, Nagy ZP, Abdelmassih R. Uterine cavity findings and hysteroscopic interventions in patients undergoing in vitro fertilization-embryo transfer who repeatedly cannot conceive. Fertil Steril. 2003;80(6):1371-5.
[32] Demirol A, Gurgan T. Effect of treatment of intrauterine pathologies with office hysteroscopy in patients with recurrent IVF failure. Reprod Biomed Online. 2004;8(6):726.
[33] Cicinelli E, Parisi C, Galantino P, Pinto V, Barba B, Schonauer S.Cicinelli E Reliability, feasibility, and safety of minihysteroscopy with a vaginoscopic approach: experience with 6,000 cases. Fertil Steril. 2003 ;80(1):199-202. Cicinelli E . Diagnostic minihysteroscopy with vaginoscopic approach: rationale and advantages. J Minim Invasive Gynecol. 2005;12(5):396-400.)
[34] Kamel HS, Darwish AM, Mohamed SA. Comparison of transvaginal ultrasonography and vaginal sonohysterography in the detection of endometrial polyps. Acta Obstet Gynecol Scand. 2000 ;79(1):60-4.
[35] Karayalcin R, Ozcan S, Moraloglu O, Ozyer S, Mollamahmutoglu L, Batıoglu S.Results of 2500 office-based diagnostic hysteroscopies before IVF. Reprod Biomed Online. 2010 May;20(5):689-93.
[36] Fatemi HM, Kasius JC , Timmermans A, van Disseldorp J, FauserB C, P. Devroey P, Broekmans FJ. Prevalence of unsuspected uterine cavity abnormalities diagnosed by office hysteroscopy prior to *in vitro* fertilization. . *Hum. Reprod.* (2010) 25 (8): 1959-1965.
[37] Kasius JC, Broekmans FJ, Veersema S, Eijkemans MJ, van Santbrink EJ, Devroey P, Fauser BC, Fatemi HM. Observer agreement in the evaluation of the uterine cavity by hysteroscopy prior to in vitro fertilization. Hum Reprod. 2011 Apr;26(4):801-7.
[38] Pundir J, El Toukhy T. Uterine cavity assessment prior to IVF. Womens Health (Lond Engl). 2010 Nov;6(6):841-7; quiz 847-8.

[39] Darwish AM, Youssef AA. Screening sonohysterography in infertility.Gynecol Obstet Invest. 48(1):43-7,1999.

[40] Kamel HS, Darwish AM, Mohamed SA. Comparison of transvaginal ultrasonography and vaginal sonohysterography in the detection of endometrial polyps. Acta Obstet Gynecol Scand. 2000 Jan;79(1):60-4.

[41] AtefM. Darwish, Ezzat H. Sayed , Safwat A. Mohammad,Ibraheem I. Mohammad, Hoida I. Hassan. Reliability of out-patient hysteroscopy in one-stop clinic for abnormal uterine bleeding. Gynecologic Surgery 2012;Volume 9, Issue 3, Page 289-295.

[42] Poncelet C, Sifer C, Hequet D, Porcher R, Wolf JP, Uzan M, Ducarme G. Hysteroscopic evaluation of endocervical and endometrial lesions observed after different procedures of embryo transfer: a prospective comparative study. Eur J Obstet Gynecol Reprod Biol. 2009 Dec;147(2):183-6.

[43] Wang XY, Li Z, A YN, Zou SH. Hysteroscopy for early abortion after IVF-ET: clinical analysis of 84 cases. Zhonghua Nan Ke Xue. 2011 Jan;17(1):52-4.

[44] Kilani Z, Shaban M, Hassan LH..Live birth after hysteroscopic-guided embryo transfer: a case report. Fertil Steril. 2009 Jun;91(6):2733.e1-2.

[45] Kitamura S, Sugiyama T, Iida E, Miyazaki T, Yoshimura Y. A New Hysteroscopic Tubal Embryo Transfer Catheter: Development and Clinical Application. Journal of Obstetrics and Gynaecology Research Volume 27, Issue 5, pages 281–284.

[46] Kamrava MM, Tran L,Hall JL. Hysteroscopic endometrial embryo delivery (HEED). In: Ectopic pregnancy- Modern Diagnosis and Management. Intech Pub Co, 2011.

[47] Kamrava, M, Yin M. Hysteroscopic Subendometrial Embryo Delivery (SEED), Mechanical Embryo Implantation. International Journal of Fertility and Sterility. Vol 4, No 1, Apr-Jun 2010, Pages: 29-34.

[48] Nalini Mahajan and Ila Gupta. Use of Versapoint to refashion the cervical canal to overcome unusually difficult embryo transfers and improve *in-vitro* fertilization-embryo transfer outcome: A case series. J Hum Reprod Sci. 2011; 4(1): 12–16.

[49] Shang Yu Huang,Chin-Jung Wang, Yung-Kuei Soong, Hsin-Shih Wang, Mei Li Wang, Chieh Yu Lin, and Chia Lin Chang. Site-specific endometrial injury improves implantation and pregnancy in patients with repeated implantation failures. Reprod Biol Endocrinol. 2011; 9: 140.

[50] Almog B, Shalom-Paz E, Dufort D, Tulandi T.Promoting implantation by local injury to the endometrium. Fertil Steril. 2010 Nov;94(6):2026-9.

[51] Ahinko-Hakamaa K, Huhtala H, Tinkanen H. The validity of air and saline hysterosalpingo-contrast sonography in tubal patency investigation before insemination treatment. European Journal of Obstetrics and Gynecology and Reproductive Biology 2007; 132, 83–87.

[52] Strandell A. The influence of hydrosalpinx on IVF and embryo transfer: a review. Hum Reprod Update 2000;6:387–95.

[53] Nackley, A.C. and Muasher, S.H. The significance of hydrosalpinx in in vitro fertilisation. Fertil Steril 1998; 69, 373–384.

[54] Camus E, Poncelet C, Goffinet F, Wainer B, Merlet F, Nisand I, et al. Pregnancy rates after in-vitro fertilization in cases of tubal infertility with and without hydrosalpinx: a meta-analysis of published comparative studies. Hum Reprod 1999;14:1243–9.
[55] Strandell A, Waldenstrom U, Nilsson L, Hamberger L. Hydrosalpinx reduces in-vitro fertilization/embryo transfer pregnancy rates. Hum Reprod 1994;9:861–3.
[56] Darwish AM, ElSamam M. Is there a role for hysteroscopic tubal occlusion of functionless hydrosalpinges prior to IVF/ICSI in modern practice. Acta Obstetricia et Gynecologica. 2007; 86: 1484_1489.
[57] A.M.Darwish, A.M.Ahmad and A.M.Mohammad. Cervical priming prior to operative hysteroscopy: a randomized comparison of laminaria versus misoprostol. Human Reproduction 2004; Vol.19, No.10 pp. 2391–2394.
[58] Peacock LM, Rock JA. Distal tubal reconstructive surgery. In: Sanfilippo JS, Levine RL, editors. Operative gynecologic endoscopy. New York: Springer-Verlag Inc; 1996. p. 182_91.
[59] Seli E, Kayisli UA, Cakmak H, Bukulmez O, Bildirici I, Guzeloglu-Kayisli O. Removal of hydrosalpinges increases endometrial leukaemia inhibitory factor (LIF) expression at the time of the implantation window. Hum Reprod. 2005;20(11):3012-7.
[60] Zeyneloglu HB, Arici A, Olive DL. Adverse effects of hydrosalpinx on pregnancy rates after in vitro fertilization embryo transfer. Fertil Steril. 1998;70:492-9.
[61] Chan LY, Chiu PY, Cheung LP, Haines CJ, Tung HF, Lau TK. A study of teratogenicity of hydrosalpinx fluid using a whole rat embryo culture model. Hum Reprod. 2003;18(5):955-8.
[62] Nackley AC, Muasher SH. The significance of hydrosalpinx in in vitro fertilisation. Fertil Steril. 1998;69:373-84.
[63] Sagoskin AW, Lessey BA, Mottla GL, Richter KS, Chetkowski RJ, Chang AS, et al. Salpingectomy or proximal tubal occlusion of unilateral hydrosalpinx increases the potential for spontaneous pregnancy. Hum Reprod. 2003; 18(12):2634-7.
[64] Ejdrup H, Bredkjær, Ziebe S, Hamid B, Zhou Y, Loft A, et al. Delivery rates after in-vitro fertilization following bilateral salpingectomy due to hydrosalpinges: a case control study. Human Reprod. 1999;/14(1):/101-5.
[65] Strandell A, Lindhard A, Waldenstro¨m U, Thorburn J, Janson PO, Hamberger L. Hydrosalpinx and IVF outcome: a prospective, randomized multicentre trial in Scandinavia on salpingectomy prior to IVF. Hum Reprod. 2001;/16(11): 2403-10.
[66] Johnson NP Mak W Sowter MC. Surgical treatment for tubal disease in women due to undergo in vitro fertilization (Cochrane Review). The Cochrane Library, Issue 2. Chichester, UK: John Wiley & Sons, Ltd; 2005.
[67] Atri M, Nazarnia S, Bret PM, Aldis AE, Kintzen G, Reinhold C. Endovaginal sonographic appearance of benign ovarian masses. RadioGraphics1994; 14:747 -76.
[68] Benjaminov O, Atri M. Sonography of the Abnormal Fallopian Tube *AJR* 2004; 183:737-742.
[69] Surrey ES, Schoolcraft WB. Laparoscopic management of hydrosalpinges before in vitro fertilization-embryo transfer: salpingectomy versus proximal tubal occlusion. Fertil Steril. 2001;/75(3):/612-7.

[70] Darwish AM, El-Samam M. Is there a role for hysteroscopic tubal occlusion of functionless hydrosalpinges prior to IVF/ICSI in modern practice. Acta Obstetricia et Gynecologica. 2007; 86: 1484-1489.

[71] Bromer JG, Arici A. Impact of uterine myomas on IVF outcome. Expert Review of Obstetrics & Gynecology 2008;3, 4,515-521.

[72] Rackow BW, Taylor HS. Submucosal uterine leiomyomas have a global effect on molecular determinants of endometrial receptivity. Fertil Steril. 2010 Apr;93(6):2027-34.

[73] Aboulghar, M.M., Al-Inany, H.G., Aboulghar, M.A., Serour, G.I., Mansour, R.T. Effect of myomectomy on the outcome of assisted reproductive technologiesMiddle East Fertility Society Journal 2004; 9 (3),263-267.

[74] Bendifallah S, Brun JL, Fernandez H. Myomectomy for infertile women: The role of surgery. J Gynecol Obstet Biol Reprod. 2011 Dec;40(8):885-901.

[75] Practice Committee of the American Society for Reproductive Medicine. Committee opinion: role of tubal surgery in the era of assisted reproductive technology. Fertil Steril. 2012 Mar;97(3):539-45.

[76] The Practice Committee of the American Society for Reproductive Medicine in Colloration with the Society of Reproductive Surgeons. Myoma and reproductive function. Fertil Steril. 2008;90:S125-30.

Chapter 3

The Use of rLH, HMG and hCG in Controlled Ovarian Stimulation for Assisted Reproductive Technologies

Micah J. Hill and Anthony M. Propst

Additional information is available at the end of the chapter

http://dx.doi.org/10.5772/50035

1. Introduction

The physiologic roles of both follicle stimulating hormone and luteinizing hormone are well established in the natural menstrual cycle. Research by Ryan and colleges in the 1960s established the concept of two different cells in the ovarian follicle, the thecal and granulosa cells, functioning in different manners to produce products of the steroid pathway, the "two cell hypothesis" (1, 2). Further work over the next two decades established the "two-cell two-gonadotropin" theory, demonstrating the action of FSH on granulosa cells and LH on thecal cells (3). Thecal cells alone were shown to express CYP17, the gene encoding for the critical enzyme in the conversion of progesterone and pregnenalone to androgens (3). Conversely, granulosa cells were demonstrated to be the cell expressing aromatase, allowing for the conversion of the androgens derived from the thecal cells to be converted to estrogens. The cooperation of both cells under the influence of both gonadotropins is essential for normal folliculogenesis and steroidogenesis in the ovary.

LH has several physiologic roles within the ovary in addition to its roll in androgen production (Figure 1). LH receptor activation leads to increases in adenylate cyclase and cAMP, resulting in increased mitochondrial transport of cholesterol necessary for steroidogeneis through upregulation of StAR (4, 5). LH activity also induces the expression of EGF-like growth factors amphiregulin and epiregulin from luteinized granulosa cells (6). These factors protect these cells from apoptosis, induce pro-survival signaling cascades, and are critical in peri-ovulatory events (6, 7). The mid-cycle LH surge causes a cascade of events leading to ovulation of the oocyte from the ovarian follicle and take the oocyte out of meiotic arrest (8). Finally, LH receptors have been demonstrated in the endometrium during the implantation window, raising a possible roll for LH in peri-implantation endometrial events

(9, 10). The specific importance of LH activity can be demonstrated in patients with LHβ or LH receptor gene mutations. Case reports of these male and female patients have demonstrated hypogonadism, infertility, pseudohermaphroditism, and amenorrhea (11-13).

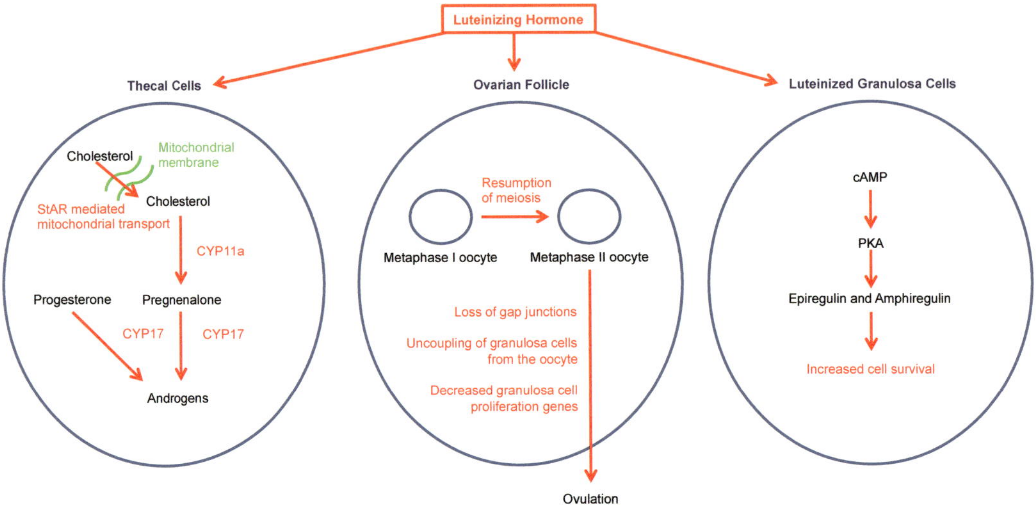

Figure 1. Key actions of LH within the ovary on the thecal cells, oocyte, and granulosa cells. Actions mediated by LH are indicated in red.

In assisted reproduction technologies (ART), the importance of LH is demonstrated clearly in hypogonadotropic hypogonadic patients. Patients with a profound lack of endogenous LH fail to undergo complete follicular maturation in the absence of exogenous LH (14, 15). Such patients require the exogenous administration of both LH and FSH to optimize reproductive outcomes (4, 16, 17). Urinary human menopausal gonadotropins were initially utilized in assisted reproductive technologies. These preparations were islolated and purified from large pools of human urine. One of the early urinary hMG products was Pergonal 75. One ampule of Pergonal 75 contained 75 international units (IU) of FSH and 75 IU of LH, which became an industry standard for ampules (18). These urinary hMG preparations contained both FSH and LH, as well as some hCG, and therefore patients were stimulated with both gonadotropins. Later advancements in monoclonal antibody technology enabled the production of urinary purified FSH and a more purified hMG, which is still used today (19, 20). Recombinant DNA technology using a mammalian cell culture system (Chinese hamster ovary cells) was used to produce recombinant human FSH, which was first licensed in 1995, and quickly replaced urinary FSH products. Recombinant human LH was later produced (18).

Despite the clear biologic importance of LH outlined in the preceding paragraphs, numerous studies have demonstrated successful ART outcomes with the use of exogenous FSH only (21, 22). A likely explanation is that LH is a very potent hormone, activating the LH receptor for adequate ovarian steroidogenesis when only 1% of LH receptors are bound (23). Even after GnRH agonist or antagonist down-regulation, a majority of patients will have LH levels > 1 IU/L, a level presumably capable of driving adequate steroidogenesis (21). While the majority of patients have adequate endogenous LH levels to have successful ART cycles without exogenous LH, the value of additional exogenous LH administration has been a matter of debate. This chapter will review the scientific evidence surrounding the administration of exogenous LH in various forms (rLH, hMG, hCG) and its affect on ART outcomes.

2. Potential mechanisms of exogenous LH benefit in ART

There are theoretical benefits of the use of exogenous LH for the oocyte and the endometrium. The putative purpose of controlled ovarian stimulation in ART is to maximize the number of oocytes retrieved. However, the evidence is clear that the addition of LH is not associated with an increase in the number of oocytes or the number of mature metaphase II oocytes (MII) retrieved. Indeed, the use of hMG has been shown to decrease the number of follicles, oocytes, and metaphase II oocytes (MII) as compared to rFSH alone (21, 22, 24-28), presumably due to the action of LH contained in hMG. This is confirmed by similar data comparing rLH plus rFSH versus rFSH alone which has shown a decrease in developing follicles and oocytes retrieved with rLH (29, 30). In the majority of these trials, the decrease was in oocytes from small to intermediate follicles, and the number of oocytes retrieved from large follicles and the number of MIIs retrieved were not different. This suggests the possibility that the use of exogenous LH activity is associated with a decreased in the development of small follicles which may have been unlikely to yield a fertilized 2PN. There appears to be no negative effect on the development of larger follicles.

In a series of *in vivo* studies evaluating the effect of LH activity on follicle growth, Filicori and colleges confirmed the findings that LH activity can decrease the growth of small follicles without impacting the continued growth and maturity of larger follicles. First, they demonstrated that the number of follicles under 10mm in size during ART stimulation positively correlated with FSH dose ($r=0.193$, $p<0.05$) but negatively correlated to LH dose ($r=0.648$, $p<0.0001$) (31). In another study, it was demonstrated that incrementally decreasing the dose of FSH from day 7 of stimulation and increasing the dose of LH resulted in a decrease in the number of follicles <10mm in size, without affecting follicles over 14mm in size (32). To evaluate if this effect was due to the decreasing FSH dose or the increasing LH dose, they performed a similar experiment where FSH was held steady at 150IU per day and patients were placed into groups of incrementally increasing LH doses. In this experiment, increasing doses of LH (in the presence of a constant dose of FSH) was again associated with a decrease in number of small follicles while not affecting the larger follicles (33). When the experiments were repeated utilizing hMG, hMG was also associated with a decrease in small follicles (34). These experiments and the results of many randomized controlled trials demonstrate that any beneficial effect of LH activity is not the result of an increase in oocyte yield.

While the number of total oocytes, especially from small follicles, appears to be diminished in ART cycles utilizing LH, the quality of those oocytes may be increased. While direct measures of oocyte quality are difficult to assess clinically, some studies have noted an increased fertilization rate in oocytes obtained from cycles stimulated with LH (24, 30). Numerous trials have also demonstrated that the addition of LH activity results in an increase in serum estradiol on the day of hCG (Figure 2), which may represent a higher quality cohort of developing follicles (22, 26, 30, 35-43). LH supplementation was demonstrated to result in lower levels of apoptosis in cumulous cells as compared to FSH stimulation only (44). Cumulous cell apoptosis has been used a marker of oocyte quality and the decrease in apoptosis with the addition of LH is consistent with its post-receptor effects through increased epiregulin and amphiregulin.

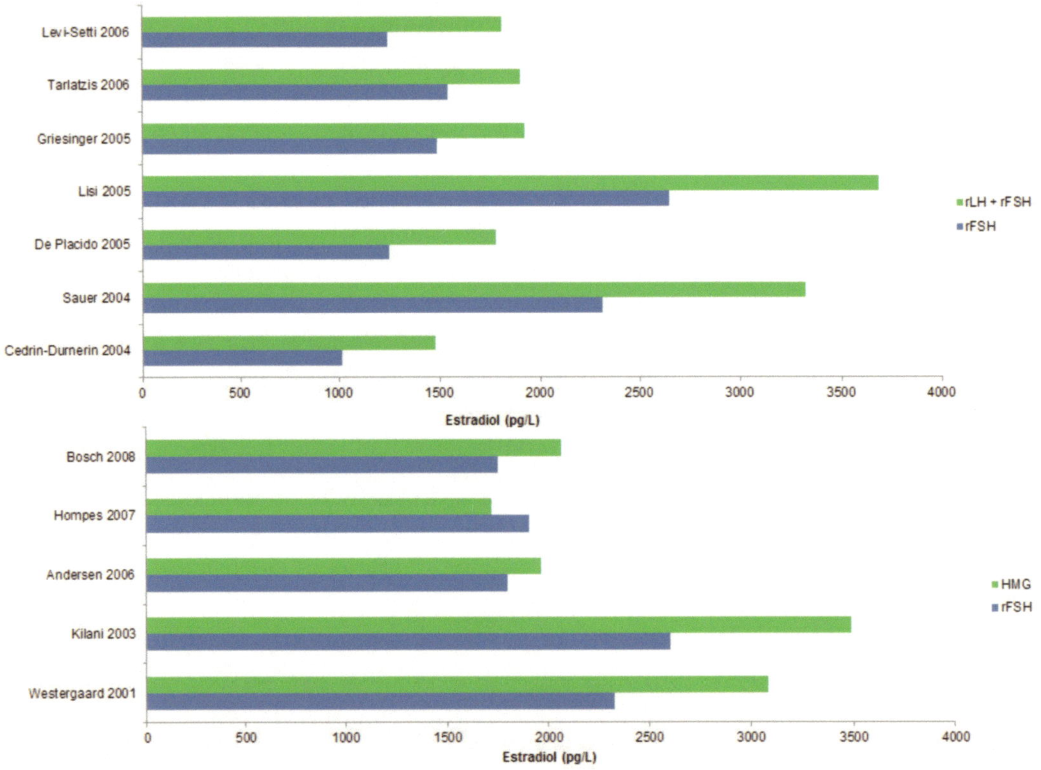

Figure 2. Randomized controlled trials demonstrating an increased estradiol level on the day of hCG with rLH (top) or hMG (bottom) as compared to rFSH alone (adapted from Hill *et al.*, 2012 (21)).

Another possible effect of LH is on the endometrium and embryo implantation. LH receptors are present in the endometrium during the window of implantation (9, 10), but whether these receptors play a direct role in embryo implantation needs further investigation. An indirect effect on the endometrium has been proposed via decreased premature progesterone secretion (24, 45). There is a growing body of evidence to suggest that prematurely elevated progesterone levels on the day of hCG have a negative impact on embryo implantation without affecting embryo quality (46-51). The evidence that this is an endometrial effect is supported by studies in oocyte donor cycles, where elevation of progesterone in the donor is not associated with decreased implantation in the recipient (52). Progesterone is necessary for endometrial development and embryo implantation. However, premature rises in progesterone can advance the development of the endometrium and lead to asynchrony with the embryo development (46, 51, 53). FSH drives the conversion of cholesterol to progesterone but lacks CYP17 to further convert progesterone to androgens (54, 55). LH stimulates CYP17 in thecal cells to further convert the progesterone to androgens, which are subsequently aromatized in the granulosa cell (3). Under the two-cell two gonadotropin model, LH is protective of premature progesterone elevations prior to luteinization (24, 45) (Figure 3). Further investigation is needed to determine if exogenous LH administration is protective for the endometrium.

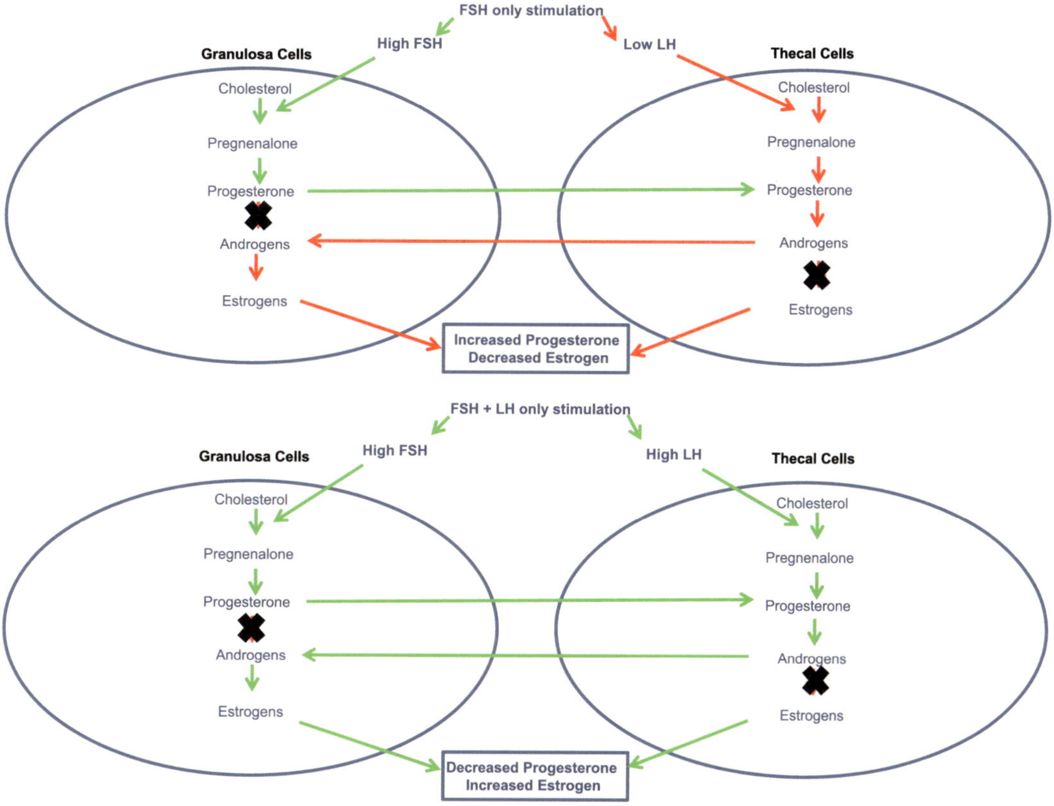

Figure 3. Model demonstrating a possible mechanism by which the administration of exogenous LH decreases premature rises in serum progesterone. FSH stimulates granulosa cells to convert cholesterol to progesterone. Lacking CYP17, the granulosa cells cannot convert progesterone to androgens and thus progesterone is secreted from the cells. In the absence of adequate LH levels, this progesterone is secreted into the circulation where it can advance the endometrium prematurely. In the presence of adequate LH levels, the progesterone is converted into androgens by CYP17 in the thecal cells. The androgens are then taken up by the granulosa cells and converted to estrogens. In this model exogenous LH protects the endometrium from exposure to premature progesterone rises. Green arrows represent increased action. Red arrows represent decreased action.

There is evidence to suggest that suppressed LH levels in women during ART stimulation can have negative effects (Figure 4). Depending on the study, adverse outcomes have been demonstrated with LH below 0.5-1.2 IU/L. LH levels < 1.2 IU/L have been reported to be associated with decreased serum estradiol, poor follicular development, decreased oocyte yield, decreased high quality embryos, and lower pregnancy rates (14, 15). Below LH levels of 1IU/L, other researchers demonstrated slower follicular growth and decreased estradiol (56). Finally, LH levels < 0.5 IU/L have been associated with increased pregnancy loss, lower implantation rates, and lower live birth rates (57, 58).

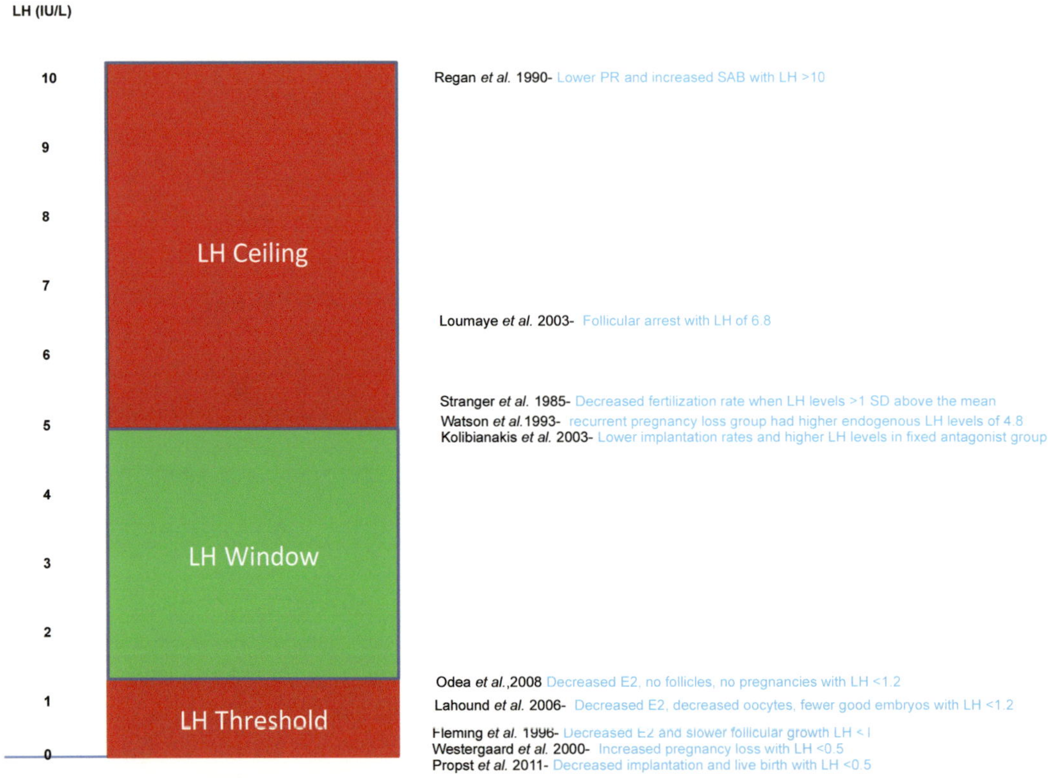

Figure 4. Demonstrates the concept of an LH window. Low LH levels have been associated with decreased poor pregnancy outcomes with levels below 0.5-1.2 IU/L, demonstrating a threshold below which low LH causes poor outcomes. High LH levels have also been associated with poor pregnancy outcomes with levels over 6.8-10 IU/L. This gives rise to the concept of a therapeutic LH window (in green) to maximize ART outcomes.

It has also been demonstrated that elevated LH levels are associated with negative ART cycle outcomes. Decreased pregnancy rates and increased spontaneous abortion were reported with LH levels above 10 IU/L (59). Increased follicular arrest, decreased fertilization, higher recurrent pregnancy loss, and lower implantation rates have all been reported in patients with higher LH levels that controls, although ceiling values were not established in these studies (56, 60-63). This evidence that too much or too little LH activity can have negative outcomes has led to the concept of an LH window (4, 61, 64). In reality, with GnRH analogues, most patients are not in danger of having elevated endogenous LH levels. Indeed, by day 6 of GnRH antagonist administration, endogenous LH levels are depressed to a mean level of 1.6 IU/L, a value much closer to the LH threshold than the ceiling (65). Similarly, long agonist protocols also suppress endogenous LH levels to a mean near 1 IU/L (66). The evidence would suggest the clinician should be more concerned with replacing an adequate LH level in patients under pituitary down-regulation and the threat of high LH levels is less prevalent.

2.1. Summary points

1. LH activity causes atresia of small follicles during ART stimulation
2. Indirect evidence suggests increased oocyte quality with LH
3. LH activity decreases oocyte yield due to a loss of these small follicle
4. LH activity increases estradiol production from follicles
5. LH activity may protect the patient from premature progesterone elevations

3. Human menopausal gonadotropin

hMG is a urinary gonadotropin preparation consisting equal activity of both LH and FSH and some hCG. It is available in highly purified forms, minimizing earlier preparation disadvantages of protein contamination leading to the risk of allergic reactions. Evaluating studies with hMG have the advantage of homogeneity. Due to the nature of hMG containing equal FSH and LH activity, all patients in the hMG group receive equal amounts of LH and FSH activity and start LH activity on the same day as the FSH activity is started. As hMG has been available for longer than rFSH, there are more studies and total data available for analysis.

When looking at intermediate outcomes and surrogate markers for ART, hMG has not been demonstrably different than rFSH for ovarian stimulation. The results are similar in the proportion of MII oocytes, the number of high quality embryos, zona pellucida morphology, and polar body evaluation (42, 67-69). Studies have also shown no benefit in the number of oocytes retrieved with hMG and indeed numerous studies have shown a small decrease in the number of oocytes retrieved (typically around 1 oocyte less per retrieval) (22, 25-28, 41, 67). In the majority of studies, the decrease in oocytes did not translate into a decrease in the number of MIIs retrieved per cycle, indicating the loss was in smaller, immature oocytes. hMG administration has been associated with higher serum and follicular fluids androgens and estrogens and lower serum progesterone levels on the day of hCG (22, 25, 41-43, 56, 70-72). It has been proposed that this more favorable endocrine milieu reflects a healthier cohort of developing follicles in hMG cycles. One study also demonstrated increasing implantation rates with increasing doses of LH supplementation (73). This dose dependent benefit of LH could be due to an increase in the quality of the oocytes retrieved or due to an endometrial effect on implantation. However, this study was small and we are not aware that the findings have been confirmed.

There is a large body of randomized controlled trials available for analysis comparing hMG to rFSH only. These trials are relatively homogenous, with similar dosing strategies and primarily GnRH agonist pituitary downregulation. These RCT have been systematically evaluated in several meta-analyses shown in Table 1 (74-78). The number of patients required to show a benefit in hMG had been calculated at over 2100 (76). This is demonstrated in a 2005 meta-analysis by Al-Inany *et al.* where 8 RCTs including 2031 ART cycles failed to show a statistically significant improvement in live birth (OR 1.18, 95%CI 0.93-1.50) although a trend to benefit may have been seen (76). When the same authors repeated a meta-analysis in 2008, there were 11 RCTs including over 2900 patients available for analysis (75). This time a significant improvement in live birth (OR 1.20, 95%CI 1.01-1.42) was demonstrated with the use of hMG versus rFSH alone (75). This data was confirmed in a separate meta-analysis by Coomarasamy *et al.* showing an improvement in live birth with hMG (OR 1.18, 95%CI 1.02-1.38) (77). Two more recent meta-analyses in 2010 each failed to show a significant improvement in live birth with the use of hMG (74, 78). However, the p values for these studies were borderline significant (0.051-0.06) and the odds ratio of pregnancy was similar to the other trials. Indeed, the last four meta-analyses had all demonstrated between a 3-4% absolute increase in pregnancy and a 10-21% relative increase in pregnancy with the use of hMG as compared to rFSH alone. These numbers translate to a NNT of approximately 32 patients with hMG to achieve one additional live birth. The clinical relevance of this number has been a matter of debate, but there is a clear statistical benefit to utilizing hMG. The majority of these source RCTs for these meta-analysis were from cycles utilizing a GnRH agonist protocols.

Author, Year	RTCs	Number of Patients	Absolute Pregnancy Benefit	Relative Pregnancy Benefit	Pregnancy OR (95% CI)
Al-Inany, 2005	8	2031	-	-	1.18 (0.93-1.50)
Al-Inany, 2008	11	2937	+3%	+21%	1.20 (1.01-1.42)
Coomarasamy, 2008	7	2159	+4%	+18%	1.18 (1.02-1.38)
Jee, 2010	5	2299	+3%	+12%	1.14 (0.98-1.33)
Lehert, 2010	16	3952	+3%	+10%	1.10 (0.97-1.25)

Table 1. Recent meta-analysis comparing hMG versus rFSH for ovarian stimulation in ART cycles.

A recent RCT published in 2012 has provided similar evidence for the benefit of hMG in GnRH antagonist cycles. Devroey *et al.* randomized 749 patients to receive either hMG or rFSH (79). There were numerous strengths to this trial: rigorously described randomization, allocation and concealment, the use of 25 clinics in 7 countries, all patients were only allowed a single blastocyst transfer, and the follow-up included live births from the fresh cycle plus subsequent frozen cycles of embryos obtained during the study. Patients in the hMG arm had higher estradiol, LH, and FSH measured in the serum on the day of hCG. There was a significant reduction in the number of oocytes retrieved in the hMG group (-1.6 oocytes per retrieval). Importantly, an absolute difference of +3% in live birth with the use of hMG in the pre-protocol analysis and +2% in the intent-to-treat analysis, although the findings did not achieve statistical significance (79). The cumulative live birth rate (fresh and frozen cycles) was 40% in the hMG group and 38% in the rFSH group. This study was in agreement with a prior publication evaluating 280 patients using a GnRH antagonist protocol with hMG or rFSH, also showing a non-significant 3% improvement in live birth rate (22). While there is not enough data to definitively conclude that hMG is beneficial in GnRH antagonist cycles, the available data shows a similar improvement to that seen in GnRH agonist cycles.

3.1. Summary points

1. hMG is a urinary derived gonadotropin formulation containing equal amounts of LH and FSH activity
2. hMG may decrease the number of oocyte retrieved by 1 oocyte per retrieval as compared to FSH
3. hMG increases live birth by 3-4% as compared to rFSH in GnRH agonist cycles
4. hMG may also increase live birth in GnRH antagonist cycles

4. Recombinant luteinizing hormone

The advent of recombinant DNA technology eventually led to the availability of recombinant LH in clinical practice (80). Urinary isolation of LH is an inefficient process, with 60-250 IU/mg of protein isolate (81). Conversely, recombinant LH contains 20,000 – 30,000 IU/mg of protein (81). The pharmacodynamics of recombinant and urinary derived LH preparations show similar clearance, half-life, and concentration curves (16, 81). The pharmacodynamics profiles of rLH are similar whether it is administered subcutaneously or intramuscular and it does not impact the pharmacodynamics of co-administered rFSH (82-84). In hypogonadotropic hypogonadal patients, a dose of 75IU of rLH has been demonstrated to promote adequate folliculogenesis when administered with FSH (85). rLH has potential advantages over the LH activity in hMG in that there is less risk of protein contamination and allergic reaction and it allows for the LH dose to be specifically adjusted without affecting the FSH dose.

There are numerous RCT evaluating rLH plus rFSH versus rFSH alone, but the data is complicated by significant heterogeneity between the trials (29, 30, 36-41, 86-95). The fact that the rLH dose can be administered at a separate starting time and doses from the rFSH dose has allowed researchers and clinicians to be more varied in the approach to rLH administration as compared to hMG. While this has allowed for the investigation of interesting protocols, it makes interpretation and meta-analysis of the data more complex. rLH has been investigated as a priming agent started up to 7 day prior to rFSH administration, as an early follicular phase agent beginning on days 1-3 of rFSH, and as a late follicular agent starting day 5-8. The dosing of rLH has also varied from 75IU to 300IU per day or as a fixed ratio to the FSH dose.

Three RCT have shown higher implantation or pregnancy rates in women receiving rLH supplementation (24, 38, 94). Patients with an inadequate response to rFSH alone have also been shown to benefit from the addition of 150IU of rLH as compared to increasing the FSH dose by 150IU (39). However, the vast majority of RCT evaluating rLH have failed to show an improvement in clinical pregnancy when compared to rFSH alone (29, 30, 36, 37, 40, 41, 86-89, 91, 92, 95). The majority of these trials were underpowered to detect for small differences in pregnancy outcomes between the study arms.

Four meta-analyses have been done to compare the outcomes of RCTs evaluating the use of rLH in ovarian stimulation (96-99). Kolibianakis *et al.* demonstrated no difference in live birth with the use of rLH, including in sub-analysis of early and mid-follicular administration or GnRH antagonist and agonist administration (97). Baruffi *et al.* did demonstrated a higher serum estradiol on the day of hCG (+514 pg/ml) and a higher number of MII oocytes retrieved (+0.88) with the use or rLH, but these differences did not translate into improve clinical pregnancy (96). In the largest meta-analysis, Mochtar *et al.* demonstrated a trend towards improved live birth with rLH, but the result did not reach statistical significance (OR 1.22, 95%CI 0.95-1.56) (98). However, pooled analysis did show an improvement in live birth for poor responders who were stimulated with rLH (OR 1.85, 95% CI1.10-3.11) (98). rLH was shown to have increased estradiol, fewer days of stimulation, and lower FSH administration in a fourth meta-analysis, although once again no improvement in pregnancy outcomes was demonstrated (99).

Author, Year	RTCs	Number of Patients	Pregnancy Odds Ratio (95% CI)
Baruffi, 2007	5	434	0.89 (0.57-1.36)
Kolibianakis, 2007	7	701	0.92 (0.65-1.31)
Mochtar, 2007	14	2612	1.22 (0.95-1.56)
Oliveira, 2007	5	1225	1.10 (0.85-1.42)

Table 2. Meta-analyses comparing rLH plus rFSH versus rFSH only.

The data from the RCT and meta-analyses evaluating rLH is similar to that of hMG in showing a reduction in the amount of FSH required for stimulation and an increase in serum estradiol. However, these data differ in that they do not show a convincing increase in pregnancy outcomes. It is possible that this is due to the smaller numbers in the rLH meta-analysis. Only the Mochtar *et al.* paper had a power similar to that of the hMG meta-analysis to detect for live birth as an outcome. The heterogeneity within the design and results of the rLH studies themselves also is associated with a decreased power to detect for pregnancy outcomes and a wide confidence interval. It is also possible that the differences seen in the meta-analyses between rLH and hMG is not only statistical, but also due to the differences in the pharmaceuticals themselves. Differences in the glycosylation of LH between urinary and recombinant preparations and the addition of hCG to urinary preparations may lead to fundamental differences in biologic action which affect clinical results.

4.1. Summary points

1. rLH increases serum estradiol
2. rLH decreases the amount of rFSH needed for ovarian stimulation
3. It is uncertain if the addition of rLH increases pregnancy outcomes in ART

5. Human chorionic gonadotropin:

hCG and LH have a significant degree of structural homology and both act on the LH receptor. hCG has a 6-8 fold affinity for the LH receptor as compared to LH only. Glycosylation additions to hCG also give it a longer half-life than LH. This has resulted in trials investigating the ability of hCG to replace LH for ovarian stimulation.

Two studies have reported the use of hCG in the early follicular phase of ovarian stimulation (100, 101). These trials and two case reports have used various dosing strategies to deliver the hCG, including 200 IU per day for four or seven days, 50 IU per day for 14 days, and 1,250 IU in a single dose on cycle day two (100-103).

In one trial, the addition of hCG resulted in significantly greater highly quality embryos (85% versus 47%) and pregnancy rates (46% versus 31%) (100). Overall, there is a lack of randomized controlled data evaluating the use of hCG from the early follicular phase, but what data is available is promising.

hCG has been evaluated as a mid-to-late cycle supplement to rFSH stimulation cycles in six trials. The dose of hCG utilized was 200IU per day in five trials and 250IU in another (104-109). All trials were initiated with rFSH only for stimulation with hCG added when the follicles were between 12-14mm in size. Five of the trials reported a significantly higher estradiol level on the day of hCG in patients randomized to receive hCG stimulation, with increases in estradiol ranging from 700-1500 pg/ml (104-107, 109). A study by Filicori *et al.* further demonstrated a significantly higher fertilization rate in patients receiving hCG versus rFSH only (74% versus 48%) (104). The remainder of the trials did not show any differences in outcomes with hCG with regards to fertilization, implantation, or pregnancy (105-107, 109). These RCT total 614 patients and demonstrate that the addition of hCG results in higher estradiol levels and at least comparable ART outcomes to rFSH stimulation only.

In a retrospective analysis, Van Horne *et al.* demonstrated that the addition of daily hCG (50-100 IU per day) to a rFSH only stimulation protocol resulted in a decrease in average FSH administration by 1000IU per patient and resulted in a cost savings of $600 in a military healthcare facility (110). In a subsequent publication, this same group demonstrated that low dose hCG was effective at significantly improving implantation rates (54% vs. 19%) and live-birth rates (64% vs. 25%) in patients who had endogenous LH levels ≤ 0.5 IU/L, while it had no benefit in patients with LH levels >0.5 IU/L (58). A meta-analysis of over 1,000 patients has demonstrated that the addition of hCG to ovarian stimulation results in a decreased requirement for rFSH, leading to a cost savings with comparable outcomes (108).

A recent meta-analysis summarized the evidence on the use of hCG in ovarian stimulation (111). The analysis included 11 RCT and 1,068 ART cycles. While the conclusions were limited due to heterogeneity with the source studies, significant conclusions were reached. It was demonstrated that the total dose of FSH was decreased by over 800 IU in patients who were supplemented with hCG. The use of hCG resulted in a small decrease in the number of MII oocytes retrieved (WMD -0.30, 95%CI -0.44 to -.66) (111). This data is consistent with the effect of LH on follicular growth discussed earlier in the chapter and a reduction of 0.3 oocytes per patient may be of small clinical impact. In analysis of 3 of trials reporting on early follicular phase hCG administration, there was no demonstrable benefit in clinical pregnancy. However, analysis of five of the trials reporting on late follicular phase hCG demonstrated a significant benefit in clinical pregnancy (RR 1.32, 95%CI 1.06-1.64).

5.1. Summary points

1. hCG can be used to provide LH action
2. 50-200 IU per day is an appropriate hCG dose
3. hCG supplementation decreases FSH requirement and ART cycle cost
4. hCG supplementation when the lead follicle is 12-14mm improves clinical pregnancy

6. Special patient groups

The use of rLH has been evaluated specifically in patients of advanced reproductive age, defined as 35 years of age and older in most studies. Eight RCT trials have compared rLH with rFSH versus rFSH stimulation only in this patient population (24, 29, 41, 88, 91, 93, 94). None of the trials reported a significant difference in oocytes retrieved with rLH. One trial reported a significant decrease in MII oocytes retrieved (5.5 versus 6.9) per patient with the use of rLH (29). The majority of the trials were small and no differences in outcomes were demonstrated with the use of rLH. The largest trial published by Bosch *et al.* enrolled 720 total patients (24). In patients 35 years old and younger, there was no benefit to rLH administration. However, in the advanced reproductive age group, there was a significantly increased fertilization rate (68% versus 61%) and implantation rate (26.7% versus 18.6%) with the use of rLH (24). There was a trend towards increased clinical pregnancy in the patients of advanced reproductive age who were supplemented with rLH (33.5 versus 25.3, p=0.09) (24).

A meta-analysis by Hill *et al*. evaluated seven of these trials (45). In that analysis, there was a significant increase in implantation (OR 1.36, 95%CI 1.05-1.78) and in clinical pregnancy (OR 1.37, 95%CI 1.03-1.83) with the use of rLH (45). While the smaller trials have been underpowered to detect important clinical outcomes such as implantation and clinical pregnancy, both the largest trial and the meta-analysis suggest a clinical benefit to including rLH in the ovarian stimulation of patients with advanced reproductive age.

It has also been suggested that poor responders will benefit from the addition of LH. A common approach to increase LH in poor responders involves the use of the microdose flare protocol. This protocol avoids the profound suppression of endogenous LH and FSH in the early follicular phase normally achieved with long luteal downregulation protocols. Scott and Novat's initial investigation of the microdose flare found it to have higher peak estradiol, more mature follicles and more mature oocytes than a traditional agonist protocol (112). While this protocol represents a well-established approach to increasing endogenous LH and FSH, randomized controlled trials have been small and inconclusive on whether this protocol increases live birth rates (113-116). One RCT did not show any benefit to adding either rLH or low-dose rHCG to a microdose flare protocol for poor responders (117). A Cochrane review has suggested that poor responders may benefit from the addition of rLH (98). In this meta-analysis there was a marked increase in live birth with the use of rLH (OR 1.85, 95%CI 1.10-3.11) (98).

6.1. Summary points

1. rLH increases implantation and clinical pregnancy in patients 35 years and older
2. rLH increases live birth in poor responders

7. Conclusion

The action of LH is vital to both natural and assisted human reproduction. Normogonadotropic patients often have adequate endogenous LH levels, even after GnRH analogue pituitary downregulation, to have successful assisted reproduction with FSH stimulation alone. However, the addition of LH activity to ovarian stimulation has been demonstrated to improve the odds of achieving a live birth. We find the 3-4% improvement in live birth with the use of LH activity to be clinically relevant. The inclusion of LH in the stimulation of poor responders and women thirty-five and older has been shown to improve ART outcomes. Since there are currently no proven methods to determine which patients will benefit most from the addition of LH, we recommend clinicians consider some form of LH activity in the ovarian stimulation of all patients.

Author details

Micah J. Hill

Program in Reproductive and Adult Endocrinology, Eunice Kennedy Shriver National Institute of Child Health and Human Development, National Institutes of Health, Bethesda, MD, USA

Anthony M. Propst

Uniformed Services University of the Health Sciences, Department of Obstetrics and Gynecology, Bethesda, MD, USA

Acknowledgement

The views expressed in this manuscript are those of the authors and do not reflect the official policy or position of the Department of the Army, Department of Air Force, Department of Defense, or the U. S. Government.

This research was supported, in part, by Intramural research program of the Program in Reproductive and Adult Endocrinology, NICHD, NIH.

8. References

[1] Ryan KJ, Petro Z. Steroid biosynthesis by human ovarian granulosa and thecal cells. Journal of Clinical Endocrinology & Metabolism. 1966;26(1):46-52.

[2] Ryan KJ, Petro Z, Kaiser J. Steroid formation by isolated and recombined ovarian granulosa and thecal cells. Journal of Clinical Endocrinology & Metabolism. 1968;28(3):355-8

[3] Hillier SG, Whitelaw PF, Smyth CD. Follicular estrogen synthesis - the 2-cell, 2-gonadotropin model revisited. Molecular and Cellular Endocrinology. 1994 Apr;100(1-2):51-4.

[4] Shoham Z. The clinical therapeutic window for luteinizing hormone in controlled ovarian stimulation. Fertility and Sterility. 2002 Jun;77(6):1170-7.

[5] Zhang GQ, Garmey JC, Veldhuis JD. Interactive stimulation by luteinizing hormone and insulin of the steroidogenic acute regulatory (StAR) protein and 17 alpha-hydroxylase/17,20-lyase (CYP17) genes in porcine theca cells. Endocrinology. 2000 Aug;141(8):2735-42.

[6] Ben-Ami I, Armon L, Freimann S, Strassburger D, Ron-El R, Amsterdam A. EGF-like growth factors as LH mediators in the human corpus luteum. Human Reproduction. 2009 Jan;24(1):176-84.

[7] Zamah AM, Hsieh M, Chen J, Vigne JL, Rosen MP, Cedars MI, et al. Human oocyte maturation is dependent on LH-stimulated accumulation of the epidermal growth factor-like growth factor, amphiregulin(dagger). Human Reproduction. 2010 Oct;25(10):2569-78.

[8] DiLuigi A, Weitzman VN, Pace MC, Siano LJ, Maier D, Mehlmann LM. Meiotic arrest in human oocytes is maintained by a Gs signaling pathway. Biology of reproduction. [Comparative Study, Research Support, N.I.H., Extramural Research Support, Non-U.S. Gov't]. 2008 Apr;78(4):667-72.

[9] Lei ZM, Reshef E, Rao CV. The expression of human chorionic-gonadotropin luteinizing-hormone receptors in human endometrial and myometrial blood-vessels. Journal of Clinical Endocrinology & Metabolism. 1992 Aug;75(2):651-9.

[10] Reshef E, Lei ZM, Rao CV, Pridham DD, Chegini N, Luborsky JL. The presence of gonadotropin receptors in nonpregnant human uterus, human placenta, fetal membranes, and decidua. Journal of Clinical Endocrinology & Metabolism. 1990 Feb;70(2):421-30.

[11] Bruysters M, Christin-Maitre S, Verhoef-Post M, Sultan C, Auger J, Faugeron I, et al. A new LH receptor splice mutation responsible for male hypogonadism with subnormal sperm production in the propositus, and infertility with regular cycles in an affected sister. Human Reproduction. 2008 Aug;23(8):1917-23.

[12] Gromoll J, Schulz A, Borta H, Gudermann T, Teerds KJ, Greschniok A, et al. Homozygous mutation within the conserved Ala-Phe-Asn-Glu-Thr motif of exon 7 of the LH receptor causes male pseudohermaphroditism. European Journal of Endocrinology. 2002 Nov;147(5):597-608.

[13] Huhtaniemi IT. LH and FSH receptor mutations and their effects on puberty. Hormone Research. [Article; Proceedings Paper]. 2002;57:35-8.

[14] Lahoud R, Al-Jefout M, Tyler J, Ryan J, Driscoll G. A relative reduction in mid-follicular LH concentrations during GnRH agonist IVF/ICSI cycles leads to lower live birth rates. Human Reproduction. 2006 Oct;21(10):2645-9.

[15] O'Dea L, O'Brien F, Currie K, Hemsey G. Follicular development induced by recombinant luteinizing hormone (LH) and follicle-stimulating hormone (FSH) in anovulatory women with LH and FSH deficiency: evidence of a threshold effect. Current Medical Research and Opinion. 2008;24(10):2785-93.

[16] Shoham Z, Smith H, Yeko T, O'Brien F, Hemsey G, O'Dea L. Recombinant LH (lutropin alfa) for the treatment of hypogonadotrophic women with profound LH deficiency: a randomized, double-blind, placebo-controlled, proof-of-efficacy study. Clinical Endocrinology. 2008 Sep;69(3):471-8.

[17] Schoot DC, Harlin J, Shoham Z, Mannaerts B, Lahlou N, Bouchard P, et al. Recombinant human follicle-stimulating-hormone and ovarian response in gonadotropin-deficient women. Human Reproduction. 1994 Jul;9(7):1237-42.

[18] Lunenfeld B. Historical perspectives in gonadotrophin therapy. Hum Reprod Update. Historical Article [Review]. 2004 Nov-Dec;10(6):453-67.

[19] Howles CM, Loumaye E, Giroud D, Luyet G. Multiple follicular development and ovarian steroidogenesis following subcutaneous administration of a highly purified urinary FSH preparation in pituitary desensitized women undergoing IVF: a multicentre European phase III study. Hum Reprod. Clinical Trial, Clinical Trial, Phase III [Multicenter Study]. 1994 Mar;9(3):424-30.

[20] van de Weijer BH, Mulders JW, Bos ES, Verhaert PD, van den Hooven HW. Compositional analyses of a human menopausal gonadotrophin preparation extracted from urine (menotropin). Identification of some of its major impurities. Reprod Biomed Online. 2003 Nov;7(5):547-57.

[21] Hill MJ, Levy G, Levens ED. Does exogenous LH in ovarian stimulation improve assisted reproduction success? An appraisal of the literature. Reproductive biomedicine online. 2012 Mar;24(3):261-71.

[22] Bosch E, Vidal C, Labarta E, Simon C, Remohi J, Pellicer A. Highly purified hMG versus recombinant FSH in ovarian hyperstimulation with GnRH antagonists--a randomized study. Human reproduction. [Randomized Controlled Trial]. 2008 Oct;23(10):2346-51.

[23] Chappel SC, Howles C. Reevaluation of the roles of luteinizing-hormone and follicle-stimulating-hormone in the ovulatory process. Human Reproduction. 1991 Oct;6(9):1206-12.

[24] Bosch E, Labarta E, Crespo J, Simon C, Remohi J, Pellicer A. Impact of luteinizing hormone administration on gonadotropin-releasing hormone antagonist cycles: an age-adjusted analysis. Fertility and sterility. [Comparative Study Randomized Controlled Trial]. 2011 Mar 1;95(3):1031-6.

[25] Balasch J, Penarrubia J, Fabregues F, Vidal E, Casamitjana R, Manau D, et al. Ovarian responses to recombinant FSH or HMG in normogonadotrophic women following pituitary desensitization by a depot GnRH agonist for assisted reproduction. Reproductive biomedicine online. 2003 2003;7(1):35-42.

[26] Hompes PGA, Broekmans FJ, Hoozemans DA, Schats R, Grp F. Effectiveness of highly purified human menopausal gonadotropin vs. recombinant follicle-stimulating hormone in first-cycle in vitro fertilization-intracytoplasmic sperm injection patients. Fertility and Sterility. 2008 Jun;89(6):1685-93.

[27] Platteau P, Andersen AN, Balen A, Devroey P, Sorensen P, Helmgaard L, et al. Similar ovulation rates, but different follicular development with highly purified menotrophin compared with recombinant FSH in WHO Group II anovulatory infertility: a randomized controlled study. Human Reproduction. 2006 Jul;21(7):1798-804.

[28] Strehler E, Abt M, El-Danasouri I, De Santo M, Sterzik K. Impact of recombinant follicle-stimulating hormone and human menopausal gonadotropins on in vitro fertilization outcome. Fertility and Sterility. 2001 Feb;75(2):332-6.

[29] Fabregues F, Creus M, Penarrubia J, Manau D, Vanrell JA, Balasch J. Effects of recombinant human luteinizing hormone supplementation on ovarian stimulation and the implantation rate in down-regulated women of advanced reproductive age. Fertility and sterility. [Comparative Study Randomized Controlled Trial Research Support, Non-U.S. Gov't]. 2006 Apr;85(4):925-31.

[30] Durnerin CI, Erb K, Fleming R, Hillier H, Hillier SG, Howles CM, et al. Effects of recombinant LH treatment on folliculogenesis and responsiveness to FSH stimulation. Human Reproduction. 2008 Feb;23(2):421-6.

[31] Filicori M, Cognigni GE, Pocognoli P, Ciampaglia W, Bernardi S. Current concepts and novel applications of LH activity in ovarian stimulation. Trends in Endocrinology and Metabolism. 2003 Aug;14(6):267-73.

[32] Filicori M, Cognigni GE, Tabarelli C, Pocognoli P, Taraborrelli S, Spettoli D, et al. Stimulation and growth of antral ovarian follicles by selective LH activity administration in women. Journal of Clinical Endocrinology & Metabolism. 2002 Mar;87(3):1156-61.

[33] Filicori M, Cognigni GE, Pocognoli P, Tabarelli C, Spettoli D, Taraborrelli S, et al. Modulation of folliculogenesis and steroidogenesis in women by graded menotrophin administration. Human Reproduction. 2002 Aug;17(8):2009-15.

[34] Filicori M, Cognigni GE, Samara A, Melappioni S, Perri T, Cantelli B, et al. The use of LH activity to drive folliculogenesis: exploring uncharted territories in ovulation induction. Human Reproduction Update. 2002 Nov-Dec;8(6):543-57.

[35] Levi-Setti PE, Cavagna M, Bulletti C. Recombinant gonadotrophins associated with GnRH antagonist (cetrorelix) in ovarian stimulation for ICSI: Comparison of r-FSH alone and in combination with r-LH. European Journal of Obstetrics Gynecology and Reproductive Biology. 2006 Jun;126(2):212-6.

[36] Tarlatzis B, Tavmergen E, Szamatowicz M, Barash A, Amit A, Levitas E, et al. The use of recombinant human LH (lutropin alfa) in the late stimulation phase of assisted reproduction cycles: a double-blind, randomized, prospective study. Human Reproduction. 2006 Jan;21(1):90-4.

[37] Griesinger G, Schultze-Mosgau A, Dafopoulos K, Schroeder A, Schroer A, von Otte S, et al. Recombinant luteinizing hormone supplementation to recombinant follicle-stimulating hormone induced ovarian hyperstimulation in the GnRH-antagonist multiple-dose protocol. Human Reproduction. 2005 May;20(5):1200-6.

[38] Lisi F, Rinaldi L, Fishel S, Caserta D, Lisi R, Campbell A. Evaluation of two doses of recombinant luteinizing hormone supplementation in an unselected group of women undergoing follicular stimulation for in vitro fertilization. Fertility and Sterility. 2005 Feb;83(2):309-15.

[39] De Placido G, Alviggi C, Perino A, Strina I, Lisi F, Fasolino A, et al. Recombinant human LH supplementation versus recombinant human FSH (rFSH) step-up protocol during controlled ovarian stimulation in normogonadotrophic women with initial inadequate ovarian response to rFSH. A multicentre, prospective, randomized controlled trial. Human Reproduction. 2005 Feb;20(2):390-6.

[40] Sauer MV, Thornton MH, Schoolcraft W, Frishman GN. Comparative efficacy and safety of cetrorelix with or without mid-cycle recombinant LH and leuprolide acetate for inhibition of premature LH surges in assisted reproduction. Reproductive Biomedicine Online. 2004 Nov;9(5):487-93.

[41] Nyboeandersen A, Humaidan P, Fried G, Hausken J, Antila L, Bangsboll S, et al. Recombinant LH supplementation to recombinant FSH during the final days of controlled ovarian stimulation for in vitro fertilization. A multicentre, prospective, randomized, controlled trial. Human reproduction. [Multicenter Study Randomized Controlled Trial Research Support, Non-U.S. Gov't]. 2008 Feb;23(2):427-34.

[42] Kilani Z, Dakkak A, Ghunaim S, Cognigni GE, Tabarelli C, Parmegiani L, et al. A prospective, randomized, controlled trial comparing highly purified hMG with recombinant FSH in women undergoing ICSI: ovarian response and clinical outcomes. Human Reproduction. 2003 Jun;18(6):1194-9.

[43] Westergaard LG, Erb K, Laursen SB, Rex S, Rasmussen PE. Human menopausal gonadotropin versus recombinant follicle-stimulating hormone in normogonadotropic women down-regulated with a gonadotropin-releasing hormone agonist who were undergoing in vitro fertilization and intracytoplasmic sperm injection: a prospective randomized study. Fertility and Sterility. 2001 Sep;76(3):543-9.

[44] Ruvolo G, Bosco L, Pane A, Morici G, Cittadini E, Roccheri MC. Lower apoptosis rate in human cumulus cells after administration of recombinant luteinizing hormone to women undergoing ovarian stimulation for in vitro fertilization procedures. Fertility and Sterility. 2007 Mar;87(3):542-6.

[45] Hill MJ, Levens ED, Levy G, Ryan ME, Csokmay JM, Decherney AH, et al. The use of recombinant luteinizing hormone in patients undergoing assisted reproductive techniques with advanced reproductive age: a systematic review and meta-analysis. Fertility and sterility. 2012 Feb 24.

[46] Bosch E, Labarta E, Crespo J, Simon C, Remohi J, Jenkins J, et al. Circulating progesterone levels and ongoing pregnancy rates in controlled ovarian stimulation cycles for in vitro fertilization: analysis of over 4000 cycles. Human Reproduction. 2010 Aug;25(8):2092-100.

[47] Bosch E, Valencia W, Escudero E, Crespo J, Simon C, Remohi J, et al. Premature luteinization during gonadotropin-releasing hormone antagonist cycles and its relationship with in vitro fertilization outcome. Fertility and Sterility. 2003 Dec;80(6):1444-9.

[48] Fanchin R, Deziegler D, Taieb J, Hazout A, Frydman R. Premature elevation of plasma progesterone alters pregnancy rates of invitro fertilization and embryo transfer. Fertility and Sterility. 1993 May;59(5):1090-4.

[49] Fanchin R, Hourvitz A, Olivennes F, Taieb J, Hazout A, Frydman R. Premature progesterone elevation spares blastulation but not pregnancy rates in in vitro fertilization with coculture. Fertility and Sterility. 1997 Oct;68(4):648-52.

[50] Fanchin R, Righini C, Olivennes F, Ferreira AL, deZiegler D, Frydman R. Consequences of premature progesterone elevation on the outcome of in vitro fertilization: insights into a controversy. Fertility and Sterility. 1997 Nov;68(5):799-805.

[51] Fanchin R, Righini C, Olivennes F, Taieb J, de Ziegler D, Frydman R. Computerized assessment of endometrial echogenicity: clues to the endometrial effects of premature progesterone elevation. Fertility and Sterility. 1999 Jan;71(1):174-81.

[52] Melo MAB, Meseguer M, Garrido N, Bosch E, Pellicer A, Remohi J. The significance of premature luteinization in an oocyte-donation programme. Human Reproduction. 2006 Jun;21(6):1503-7.

[53] Bourgain C, Devroey P. The endometrium in stimulated cycles for IVF. Human Reproduction Update. 2003 Dec;9(6):515-22.

[54] Palermo R. Differential actions of FSH and LH during folliculogenesis. Reproductive Biomedicine Online. 2007 Sep;15(3):326-37.

[55] Voutilainen R, Tapanainen J, Chung BC, Matteson KJ, Miller WL. Hormonal-regulation of p450scc (20,22-desmolase) and p450c17 (17-alpha-hydroxylase-17,20-lyase) in cultured human granulosa-cells. Journal of Clinical Endocrinology & Metabolism. 1986 Jul;63(1):202-7.

[56] Fleming R, Chung CC, Yates RWS, Coutts JRT. Purified urinary follicle stimulating hormone induces different hormone profiles compared with menotrophins, dependent upon the route of administration and endogenous luteinizing hormone activity. Human Reproduction. 1996 Sep;11(9):1854-8.

[57] Westergaard LG, Laursen SB, Andersen CY. Increased risk of early pregnancy loss by profound suppression of luteinizing hormone during ovarian stimulation in normogonadotrophic women undergoing assisted reproduction. Human Reproduction. 2000 May;15(5):1003-8.

[58] Propst AM, Hill MJ, Bates GW, Palumbo M, Van Horne AK, Retzloff MG. Low-dose human chorionic gonadotropin may improve in vitro fertilization cycle outcomes in patients with low luteinizing hormone levels after gonadotropin-releasing hormone antagonist administration. Fertil Steril. Comparative Study [Research Support, N.I.H., Intramural]. 2011 Oct;96(4):898-904.

[59] Regan L, Owen EJ, Jacobs HS. Hypersecretion of luteinizing-hormone, infertility, and miscarriage. Lancet. 1990 Nov;336(8724):1141-4.

[60] Stanger JD, Yovich JL. Reduced in-vitro fertilization of human oocytes from patients with raised basal luteinizing hormone levels during the follicular phase. Br J Obstet Gynaecol. 1985 Apr;92(4):385-93.

[61] Loumaye E, Engrand P, Shoham Z, Hillier SG, Baird DT. Clinical evidence for an LH ceiling? Human Reproduction. 2003 Dec;18(12):2719-20.

[62] Loumaye E, Engrand P, Shoham Z, Hillier SG, Baird DT, Recombinant LHSG. Clinical evidence for an LH 'ceiling' effect induced by administration of recombinant human LH during the late follicular phase of stimulated cycles in World Health Organization type I and type II anovulation. Human Reproduction. 2003 Feb;18(2):314-22.

[63] Watson H, Kiddy DS, Hamilton-Fairley D, Scanlon MJ, Barnard C, Collins WP, et al. Hypersecretion of luteinizing hormone and ovarian steroids in women with recurrent early miscarriage. Hum Reprod. 1993 Jun;8(6):829-33.

[64] Fischer R. Understanding the role of LH: myths and facts. Reprod Biomed Online. 2007 Oct;15(4):468-77.

[65] Mannaerts B, Devroey P, Abyholm T, Diedrich K, Hillensjo T, Hedon B, et al. A double-blind, randomized, dose-finding study to assess the efficacy of the gonadotrophin-releasing hormone antagonist ganirelix (Org 37462) to prevent premature luteinizing hormone surges in women undergoing ovarian stimulation with recombinant follicle stimulating hormone (Puregon((R))). Human Reproduction. 1998 Nov;13(11):3023-31.

[66] Manna C, Rahman A, Sbracia M, Pappalardo S, Mohamed EI, Linder R, et al. Serum luteinizing hormone, follicle-stimulating hormone and oestradiol pattern in women undergoing pituitary suppression with different gonadotrophin-releasing hormone analogue protocols for assisted reproduction. Gynecological Endocrinology. 2005 Apr;20(4):188-94.

[67] Jansen CAM, van Os HC, Out HJ, Bennink H. A prospective randomized clinical trial comparing recombinant follicle stimulating hormone (Puregon) and human menopausal gonadotrophins (Humegon) in non-down-regulated in-vitro fertilization patients. Human Reproduction. 1998 Nov;13(11):2995-9.

[68] Ng EHY, Lau EYL, Yeung WSB, Ho PC. HMG is as good as recombinant human FSH in terms of oocyte and embryo quality: a prospective randomized trial. Human Reproduction. 2001 Feb;16(2):319-25.

[69] Rashidi BH, Sarvi F, Tehrani ES, Zayeri F, Movahedin M, Khanafshar N. The effect of HMG and recombinant human FSH on oocyte quality: a randomized single-blind clinical trial. European Journal of Obstetrics & Gynecology and Reproductive Biology. 2005 Jun 1;120(2):190-4.

[70] Fleming R, Jenkins J. The source and implications of progesterone rise during the follicular phase of assisted reproduction cycles. Reproductive Biomedicine Online. 2010 Oct;21(4):446-9.

[71] Smitz J, Andersen AN, Devroey P, Arce JC. Endocrine profile in serum and follicular fluid differs after ovarian stimulation with HP-hMG or recombinant FSH in IVF patients. Human Reproduction. 2007 Mar;22(3):676-87.

[72] Diedrich K, Devroey P, Engels S, Quartarolo JP, Hiller KF, Rudolf K, et al. Efficacy and safety of highly purified menotropin versus recombinant follicle-stimulating hormone in in vitro fertilization/intracytoplasmic sperm injection cycles: a randomized, comparative trial. Fertility and Sterility. 2002 Sep;78(3):520-8.

[73] Gordon UD, Harrison RF, Fawzy M, Hennelly B, Gordon AC. A randomized prospective assessor-blind evaluation of luteinizing hormone dosage and in vitro fertilization outcome. Fertility and Sterility. 2001 Feb;75(2):324-31.

[74] Lehert P, Schertz JC, Ezcurra D. Recombinant human follicle-stimulating hormone produces more oocytes with a lower total dose per cycle in assisted reproductive technologies compared with highly purified human menopausal gonadotrophin: a meta-analysis. Reproductive biology and endocrinology : RB&E. Comparative Study Meta-Analysis [Review]. 2010;8:112.

[75] Al-Inany HG, Abou-Setta AM, Aboulghar MA, Mansour RT, Serour GI. Efficacy and safety of human menopausal gonadotrophins versus meta-analysis recombinant FSH: a mate-analysis. Reproductive Biomedicine Online. 2008 Jan;16(1):81-8.

[76] Al-Inany H, Aboulghar MA, Mansour RT, Serour GI. Ovulation induction in the new millennium: Recombinant follicle-stimulating hormone versus human menopausal gonadotropin. Gynecological Endocrinology. 2005 Mar;20(3):161-9.

[77] Coomarasamy A, Afnan M, Cheema D, van der Veen F, Bossuyt PMM, van Wely M. Urinary hMG versus recombinant FSH for controlled ovarian hyperstimulation following an agonist long down-regulation protocol in IVF or ICSI treatment: a systematic review and meta-analysis. Human Reproduction. 2008 Feb;23(2):310-5.

[78] Jee BC, Suh CS, Kim YB, Kim SH, Moon SY. Clinical efficacy of highly purified hMG versus recombinant FSH in IVF/ICSI cycles: a meta-analysis. Gynecologic and obstetric investigation. Comparative Study Meta-Analysis [Review]. 2010;70(2):132-7.

[79] Devroey P, Pellicer A, Nyboe Andersen A, Arce JC. A randomized assessor-blind trial comparing highly purified hMG and recombinant FSH in a GnRH antagonist cycle with compulsory single-blastocyst transfer. Fertility and sterility. 2012 Mar;97(3):561-71.

[80] De Leo V, Musacchio MC, Di Sabatino A, Tosti C, Morgante G, Petraglia F. Present and Future of Recombinant Gonadotropins in Reproductive Medicine. Current Pharmaceutical Biotechnology. 2012 Mar;13(3):379-91.

[81] Porchet HC, Lecotonnec JY, Neuteboom B, Canali S, Zanolo G. Pharmacokinetics OF recombinant human luteinizing-hormone after intravenous, intramuscular, and subcutaneous administration in monkeys and comparison with intravenous administration of pituitary human luteinizing-hormone. Journal of Clinical Endocrinology & Metabolism. 1995 Feb;80(2):667-73.

[82] le Cotonnec JY, Loumaye E, Porchet HC, Beltrami V, Munafo A. Pharmacokinetic and pharmacodynamic interactions between recombinant human luteinizing hormone and recombinant human follicle-stimulating hormone. Fertility and Sterility. 1998 Feb;69(2):201-9.

[83] le Cotonnec JY, Porchet HC, Beltrami V, Munafo A. Clinical pharmacology of recombinant human luteinizing hormone: Part I. Pharmacokinetics after intravenous administration to healthy female volunteers and comparison with urinary human luteinizing hormone. Fertility and Sterility. 1998 Feb;69(2):189-94.

[84] le Cotonnec JY, Porchet HC, Beltrami V, Munafo A. Clinical pharmacology of recombinant human luteinizing hormone: Part II. Bioavailability of recombinant human luteinizing hormone assessed with an immunoassay and an in vitro bioassay. Fertility and Sterility. 1998 Feb;69(2):195-200.

[85] Recombinant human luteinizing hormone (LH) to support recombinant human follicle-stimulating hormone (FSH)-induced follicular development in LH- and FSH-deficient anovulatory women: a dose-finding study. The European Recombinant Human LH Study Group. J Clin Endocrinol Metab. 1998 May;83(5):1507-14.

[86] Balasch J, Creus M, Fabregues F, Civico S, Carmona F, Puerto B, et al. The effect of exogenous luteinizing hormone (LH) on oocyte viability: Evidence from a comparative study using recombinant human follicle-stimulating hormone (FSH) alone or in combination with recombinant LH for ovarian stimulation in pituitary-suppressed women undergoing assisted reproduction. Journal of Assisted Reproduction and Genetics. 2001 May;18(5):250-6.

[87] Balasch J, Miro F, Burzaco I, Casamitjana R, Civico S, Ballesca JL, et al. The role of luteinizing-hormone in human follicle development and oocyte fertility - evidence from in-vitro fertilization in a woman with long-standing hypogonadotropic hypogonadism and using recombinant human follicle-stimulating-hormone. Human Reproduction. 1995 Jul;10(7):1678-83.

[88] Barrenetxea G, Agirregoikoa JA, Jimenez MR, de Larruzea AL, Ganzabal T, Carbonero K. Ovarian response and pregnancy outcome in poor-responder women: a randomized controlled trial on the effect of luteinizing hormone supplementation on in vitro fertilization cycles. Fertility and sterility. [Randomized Controlled Trial]. 2008 Mar;89(3):546-53.

[89] Cedrin-Durnerin I, Grange-Dujardin D, Laffy A, Parneix I, Massin N, Galey J, et al. Recombinant human LH supplementation during GnRH antagonist administration in IVF/ICSI cycles: a prospective randomized study. Human Reproduction. 2004 Sep;19(9):1979-84.

[90] De Placido G, Alviggi C, Mollo A, Strina I, Ranieri A, Alviggi E, et al. Effects of recombinant LH (rLH) supplementation during controlled ovarian hyperstimulation (COH) in normogonadotrophic women with an initial inadequate response to recombinant FSH (rFSH) after pituitary downregulation. Clinical Endocrinology. 2004 May;60(5):637-43.

[91] Humaidan P, Bungum M, Bungum L, Andersen CY. Effects of recombinant LH supplementation in women undergoing assisted reproduction with GnRH agonist

down-regulation and stimulation with recombinant FSH: an opening study. Reproductive Biomedicine Online. 2004 Jun;8(6):635-43.

[92] Kovacs P, Kovats T, Kaali SG. Results with early follicular phase recombinant luteinizing hormone supplementation during stimulation for in vitro fertilization. Fertility and Sterility. 2010 Jan 15;93(2):475-9.

[93] Marrs R, Meldrum D, Muasher S, Schoolcraft W, Werlin L, Kelly E. Randomized trial to compare the effect of recombinant human FSH (follitropin alfa) with or without recombinant human LH in women undergoing assisted reproduction treatment. Reproductive Biomedicine Online. 2004 Feb;8(2):175-82.

[94] Matorras R, Prieto B, Exposito A, Mendoza R, Crisol L, Herranz P, et al. Mid-follicular LH supplementation in women 35-39 years undergoing ICSI cycles: a randomized controlled study. Reproductive Biomedicine Online. 2009 Dec;19(6):879-87.

[95] Sills ES, Levy DP, Moomjy M, McGee M, Rosenwaks Z. A prospective, randomized comparison of ovulation induction using highly purified follicle-stimulating hormone alone and with recombinant human luteinizing hormone in in-vitro fertilization. Human Reproduction. 1999 Sep;14(9):2230-5.

[96] Baruffi R, Mauri AL, Petersen C, Felipe V, Martins A, Cornicelli J, et al. Recombinant LH supplementation to recombinant FSH during induced ovarian stimulation in the GnRH-antagonist protocol: a meta-analysis. Reproductive Biomedicine Online. 2007 Jan;14(1):14-25.

[97] Kolibianakis EM, Kalogeropoulou L, Griesinger G, Papanikolaou EG, Papadimas J, Bontis J, et al. Among patients treated with FSH and GnRH analogues for in vitro fertilization, is the addition of recombinant LH associated with the probability of live birth? A systematic review and meta-analysis. Human Reproduction Update. 2007 Sep-Oct;13(5):445-52.

[98] Mochtar MH, Van der V, Ziech M, van Wely M. Recombinant Luteinizing Hormone (rLH) for controlled ovarian hyperstimulation in assisted reproductive cycles. Cochrane Database of Systematic Reviews. 2007(2).

[99] Oliveira JBA, Mauri AL, Petersen CG, Martins AMC, Cornicelli J, Cavanha M, et al. Recombinant luteinizing hormone supplementation to recombinant follicle-stimulation hormone during induced ovarian stimulation in the GnRH-agonist protocol: A meta-analysis. Journal of Assisted Reproduction and Genetics. 2007 Mar;24(2-3):67-75.

[100] Beretsos P, Partsinevelos GA, Arabatzi E, Drakakis P, Mavrogianni D, Anagnostou E, et al. "hCG priming" effect in controlled ovarian stimulation through a long protocol. Reproductive Biology and Endocrinology. 2009 Aug 31;7.

[101] Drakakis P, Loutradis D, Beloukas A, Sypsa V, Anastasiadou V, Kalofolias G, et al. Early hCG addition to rFSH for ovarian stimulation in IVF provides better results and the cDNA copies of the hCG receptor may be an indicator of successful stimulation. Reproductive Biology and Endocrinology. 2009 Oct 13;7.

[102] Filicori M, Cognigni GE, Taraborrelli S, Spettoli D, Ciampaglia W, de Fatis CT. Low-dose human chorionic gonadotropin therapy can improve sensitivity to exogenous follicle-stimulating hormone in patients with secondary amenorrhea. Fertility and Sterility. 1999 Dec;72(6):1118-20.

[103] Lossl K, Andersen CY, Loft A, Freiesleben NLC, Bangsboll S, Andersen AN. Short-term androgen priming by use of aromatase inhibitor and hCG before controlled ovarian stimulation for IVF. A randomized controlled trial. Human Reproduction. 2008 Aug;23(8):1820-9.
[104] Filicori M, Cognigni GE, Gamberini E, Parmegiani L, Troilo E, Roset B. Efficacy of low-dose human chorionic gonadotropin alone to complete controlled ovarian stimulation. Fertility and Sterility. 2005 Aug;84(2):394-401.
[105] Koichi K, Yukiko N, Shima K, Sachiko S. Efficacy of low-dose human chorionic gonadotropin (hCG) in a GnRH antagonist protocol. Journal of Assisted Reproduction and Genetics. 2006 May;23(5):223-8.
[106] Serafini P, Yadid I, Motta ELA, Alegretti JR, Fioravanti J, Coslovsky M. Ovarian stimulation with daily late follicular phase administration of low-dose human chorionic gonadotropin for in vitro fertilization: a prospective, randomized trial. Fertility and Sterility. 2006 Oct;86(4):830-8.
[107] Gomes MKO, Vieira CS, Moura MD, Manetta LA, Leite SP, Reis RM, et al. Controlled ovarian stimulation with exclusive FSH followed by stimulation with hCG alone, FSH alone or hMG. European Journal of Obstetrics Gynecology and Reproductive Biology. 2007 Jan;130(1):99-106.
[108] Kosmas IP, Zikopoulos K, Georgiou I, Paraskevaidis E, Blockeel C, Tournaye H, et al. Low-dose HCG may improve pregnancy rates and lower OHSS in antagonist cycles: a meta-analysis. Reproductive Biomedicine Online. 2009 Nov;19(5):619-30.
[109] Kyono K, Fuchinoue K, Nakajo Y, Yagi A, Sasaki K. A prospective randomized study of three ovulation induction protocols for IVF: GnRH agonist versus antagonist with and without low dose hCG. Fertility and Sterility. 2004 Sep;82:S31-S.
[110] Propst AM, Bates GW, Robinson RD, Arthur NJ, Martin JE, Neal GS. A randomized controlled trial of increasing recombinant follicle-stimulating hormone after initiating a gonadotropin-releasing hormone antagonist for in vitro fertilization-embryo transfer. Fertility and Sterility. 2006 Jul;86(1):58-63.
[111] Checa MA, Espinos JJ, Requena A. Efficacy and safety of human chorionic gonadotropin for follicular phase stimulation in assisted reproduction: a systematic review and meta-analysis. Fertility and sterility. 2012 Mar 29.
[112] Scott RT, Navot D. Enhancement of ovarian responsiveness with microdoses of gonadotropin-releasing-hormone agonist during ovulation induction for in-vitro fertilization. Fertility and Sterility. 1994 May;61(5):880-5.
[113] Kahraman K, Berker B, Atabekoglu CS, Sonmezer M, Cetinkaya E, Aytac R, et al. Microdose gonadotropin-releasing hormone agonist flare-up protocol versus multiple dose gonadotropin-releasing hormone antagonist protocol in poor responders undergoing intracytoplasmic sperm injection-embryo transfer cycle. Fertility and Sterility. 2009 Jun;91(6):2437-44.
[114] Demirol A, Gurgan T. Microdose flare versus antagonist for poor responders Reply. Fertility and Sterility. 2010 May;93(7):E36-E.
[115] Akman MA, Erden HF, Tosun SB, Bayazit N, Aksoy E, Bahceci M. Comparison of agonistic flare-up-protocol and antagonistic multiple dose protocol in ovarian

stimulation of poor responders: results of a prospective randomized trial. Human Reproduction. 2001 May;16(5):868-70.

[116] Malmusi S, La Marca A, Giulini S, Xella S, Tagliasacchi D, Marsella T, et al. Comparison of a gonadotropin-releasing hormone (GnRH) antagonist and GnRH agonist flare-up regimen in poor responders undergoing ovarian stimulation. Fertility and Sterility. 2005 Aug;84(2):402-6.

[117] Berkkanoglu M, Isikoglu M, Aydin D, Ozgur K. Clinical effects of ovulation induction with recombinant follicle-stimulating hormone supplemented with recombinant luteinizing hormone or low-dose recombinant human chorionic gonadotropin in the midfollicular phase in microdose cycles in poor responders. Fertility and Sterility. 2007 Sep;88(3):665-9.

Chapter 4

The Means of Progress in Improving the Results of *in vitro* Fertilization Based on the Identification and Correction of the Pathology of Hemostasis

Andrey Momot, Inna Lydina, Lyudmila Tsyvkina,
Oksana Borisova and Galina Serdyuk

Additional information is available at the end of the chapter

http://dx.doi.org/10.5772/52898

1. Introduction

In most developed countries the problem of infertility has acquired not only medical and sociodemographic, but also economic significance. One of the key and vigorously developing trends in modern obstetrics is aimed at overcoming this problem and requires a multidisciplinary approach. The 2010 Nobel Prize was awarded to Robert Edwards, 85-year-old British researcher and recognized the methods of assisted reproductive technologies (ARTs) which introduced a new era in human demography. ARTs are used to solve the problem of infertility; they use all treatment methods and procedures which support in vitro processing of human oocytes, sperm or embryos to become pregnant. These technologies involve in vitro fertilization (IVF) and transcervical embryo transfer, gamete intrafallopian transfer, zygote intrafallopian transfer, embryo intrafallopian transfer, gamete and embryo cryopreservation, oocyte and embryo donation, and surrogacy (Current Practices and Controversies in Assisted Reproduction. Report of.., 2001).

25 July 1978 was marked by a significant event in the history of ARTs. On that day, the first "test tube baby" was born in an obstetrics and gynecology clinic located in Oldham, North West England. This was also the birth date of modern assisted reproduction. In Russia, the first baby born by this method was delivered in 1986 in the Research Center for Obstetrics, Gynecology and Perinatology, the division of the Russian Academy of Medical Sciences. Other leading centers in Russia are "Fertimed "Center for Reproduction and Genetics (Moscow), "ART-ECO" Clinic for Reproductive Health (Moscow), "ECO" Center for the

Treatment of Infertility, LLC (Moscow), International Center for Reproductive Medicine (Saint-Petersburg), the Baltic Institute of Human Reproductology (Saint-Petersburg), etc.

2. In vitro fertilization and known reasons that reduce its efficacy

In vitro fertilization of preovulatory oocytes and transfer of cleaving embryos into the patient's uterine cavity has become the prevalent method to overcome the problem of infertility (Pioneers in in vivo Fertilisation .., 1995). The IVF method was initially devised for those women whose Fallopian tubes were removed for one reason or another. However, at present, IVF is the most effective treatment for virtually all types of infertility, including endometriosis, polycystic ovary syndrome, oocyte donation (in infertile patients with oogenesis depletion), fertilization of an egg with a single sperm in cases of virtually absolute forms of male infertility (intracytoplasmic sperm injection - ICSI), carriage of an embryo by a voluntary egg recipient when a woman cannot carry the pregnancy due to some somatic or other diseases (Maheshwari et al., 2008). Despite all achievements, the IVF pregnancy rate is comparatively low. It ranges from 25% to 30% and has not changed considerably in recent years (Nyboe Andersen et al., 2009). This rate relates to a number of diverse factors that affect the reproductive process. Implantation failure following embryo transfer is the major problem in IVF (Bischof et al., 2006; Christiansen et al., 2006). IVF failures may be caused by a variety of factors: diminished ovarian reserve, maternal and paternal age, excessive body weight, endocrine disorders in the hypothalamus-pituitary-ovary system, as well as in the suprarenal and thyroid systems, diminished endometrial receptivity, quantity and quality of transferred embryos, number of transfers, and thrombophilic disorders.

Ovarian reserve. Ovarian reserve is one of the factors that determine the efficacy of IVF (Gregory, 1998; Navot et al., 1987; Scheffer et al., 2003). Assessing the ovarian reserve, specialists draw conclusions based on the prospects of ovarian stimulation in a particular patient. Conclusions may be used to define a specific procedure and further treatment prospects, as well as to make the right choice of the ovarian stimulation scheme and the quantity of drugs of human menopausal gonadotropin or follicle-stimulating hormone (FSH), which are necessary for an adequate response. The routine method for assessing the ovarian reserve measures basal FSH level on the 3rd or 4th day of the menstrual cycle and estimates the quantity of antral follicles with ultrasonography. However, at present, the prognostic significance of ultrasonography is considered less informative, even though it reflects the quantity and quality of oocytes (Damti et al., 2008). The role of new factors capable of reflecting the functional status of the ovary in a more precise manner is under discussion. (Gregory, 1998).

Maternal and paternal age. Lintsen et al. (2007) concluded that the most important prognostic indicator to define the probability of pregnancy after IVF and ICSI is maternal age (more frequently observed positive results -in 30-year-old women, less frequently - in women under 35, and least frequently - in women over 35). Physiological process of the gradual decline of ovarian function is one of the key obstacles for the efficacy of IVF, which depends on maternal age, current condition of the ovarian reserve and to a lesser extent on chosen schemes of ovulation induction. The cases of women under 41 are treated as relatively promising, to reason the use of donated oocytes in older women (Maheshwari et al., 2008). Paternal age also affects the conception rate: it shrinks with men after 35 due to the quality of sperm to have been deteriorated by this age (Saleh et al., 2002).

Excessive body weight. Menstrual dysfunction, polycystic ovary syndrome, hyperplastic processes in endometrium, infertility, miscarriage, gestoses, fetal hypotrophies, high rate of operative deliveries make up an incomplete list of reproductive disorders typical of obese women. 40% of women seeking for treatment of infertility in medical centers have excessive body weight; over 15% of such women are obese. The IVF program is preferable to start after the patient's body weight has become normalized; therefore, patients often fail to meet the required standards (Ku et al., 2006; Lintsen et al., 2005; Mc Clamrock, 2008; Megan et al., 2008). Status of the hypothalamus-pituitary-ovary system, suprarenal and thyroid systems. Interaction of the two key pituitary hormones - FSH and luteinizing hormone (LH) - is essential for the adequate growth of follicles, as well as for the formation of viable oocytes. Studies of ovulation induction in hypogonadotropic patients showed that exogenous FSH stimulates the growth of follicles up to the preovulatory stage and its synthesis primarily depends on LH, i.e. adequate maturation of follicles takes place due to this gonadotropin. Insufficient concentration of LH disturbs paracrine mechanisms regulating granulosa cells, as well as endometrial proliferation, and results in inadequate luteal phase (Alviggi et al., 2009; Balasch et al., 1995; Hull et al., 1994). Excessive concentration of LH also negatively affects the growth of follicles to be the result of suppressed aromatase activity, accompanied by fertilization disorders, decreased pregnancy rate decrease and increased miscarriage rate (Hillier, 1994). Thus, the threshold concentration (1-10 IU/l) is optimal for adequate folliculogenesis (Howles et al., 2006). It has been noted that low estradiol level in the blood serum (<200 pmole/l) on the 3rd day of the patient's menstrual cycle is a positive prognostic indicator of successful implantation in the IVF cycle. At the same time, some reports state that basal estradiol level was not a significant indicator of ovarian response to stimulation and did not correlate with the IVF result (Friedler et al., 2005). In recent years, researchers and clinicists have given a lot of consideration to the problem of thyroid gland dysfunction in infertile women (Bellver et al., 2008). Female reproductive system consists of interrelated structural elements: hypothalamus, pituitary gland, ovaries, other endocrine glands and target organs facilitating reproductive function. Thyroid gland is a chief part of the neuroendocrinal system; it significantly affects reproductive function. The hypothalamus-pituitary-gonadal and hypothalamus-pituitary-thyroid systems are closely related due to the presence of common central regulating mechanisms. For example, the spread of thyroid gland dysfunction diagnosed at the examination in women, who seek clinical diagnosis and treatment of infertility, ranges from 2.5 to 38.3% (Lazarus & Premawardhana, 2005). In addition to gonadotropic hormones, ovarian function is determined by adrenal hormones produced under impact of ACTH. When a patient has developed any genetic defects in the enzyme systems, cortisol synthesis in adrenal glands decreases with the increase of level of ACTH followed by the increased production of androgens under normal synthesis. This condition may be typical of congenital adrenal hyperplasia. As a result of adrenal hyperandrogenism, the suppression of ovarian function takes place, which leads to the development of a number of disorders in the menstrual cycle accompanied by anovulation.

Diminished endometrial receptivity. After high-quality embryos have been transferred into the uterine cavity and all evident causes for the failure of the IVF program have been eliminated, the unsuccessful IVF cycle is regarded as a result of disorders that occurred during the embryo implantation stage. A few years ago a new term - "repeated implantation failure" - was introduced (Margalioth et al., 2006; Tan et al., 2005). Recent years have shown that, despite the selection of obviously normal embryos for the transfer, only 20% of human embryos transferred in IVF cycles have been implanted in the uterus (International Committee for Monitoring Assisted Reproductive Technology (ICMART), 2002; Nyboe Andersen et al., 2009). This condition is considered to be based on the endometrial dysfunction occurring on the mollecular-cellular level. Lately, as a result of the tendency to transfer one or two embryos inside of an uterus, the method to determine repeated implantation failure has been modified. Margalioth et al. (2006) concluded that detailed examination should be done after 3 unsuccessful IVF cycles. Thus, the main causes are the factors which diminish endometrial receptivity: anatomical defects in the uterus, chronic endometritis, non-correspondence between the endometrial thickness and the day of embryo transfer, combined gynecologic pathology (adenomyosis, uterine fibroid), somatic diseases (including autoimmune diseases), and thrombophilias (Margalioth et al., 2006; Tan et al., 2005).

Quantity of transferred embryos. Due to the absence of conventional clinical guidelines for the treatment of infertility with the IVF method, there are on-going discussions regarding the elective transfer of one embryo to patients under 40. In 2009, a mathematical model was drawn to prove that the transfer of only one embryo shall decrease the pregnancy rate by 20% (Gelbaya et al., 2009).

Embryo transfer on the stages of cleavage or blastocyst. The data obtained during the systematic review and meta-analysis (Papanikolaou et al., 2008) of 1654 patients (blastocyst transferred to 815 patients, cleaving embryo transferred to 839 patients) showed that live birth rate was higher with embryos transferred on the blastocyst stage as compared to the rate at the cleavage stage. Multiple gestation rates were the same for both study groups.

3. Data on the IVF results as affected by pathologies of hemostasis

As we have already noted, unsuccessful IVF cycles are caused by many factors, including thrombogenicity of the medical technology itself due to the high estrogen-gestagen rate and frequent presence of thrombogenic risk factors and predisposition to intravascular coagulation (thrombophilia) in women that need IVF. According to up-to-date conceptions, the term "thrombophilia" means predisposition to arterial or venous thrombosis as a result of several hereditary or acquired disorders in the systems of blood coagulation, anticoagulation, or fibrinolysis (Bates et al., 2008; Heit, 2007). We use this term in a different sense, which makes most of the described thrombophilias no more than thrombogenic risk factors that may or may not become evident during the lifespan of a human being.

According to our conceptions, thrombophilia should be detected in case of everpresent thrombosis risk factors (thromboses) or miscarriage syndrome in the individual medical history. In order to prove it, we note the fact that, according to the guidelines of the International Society on Thrombosis and Haemostasis (ISTH), diagnosis of antiphospholipid syndrome (APS) shall be considered invalid unless at least one or more clinical implications of this pathology match the results of special laboratory assays (lupus anticoagulant effects, antiphospholipid antibodies in the diagnostic titer) (Harris & Pierangeli, 2008).

Some publications indicate data on typical changes in the system of hemostasis that occurs during the IVF cycle. In particular, demonstration has shown that hormonal stimulation of the ovaries is accompanied by the increased von Willebrand factor, factors V and VIII, fibrinogen, enhanced APC resistance, and the decreased activity of principal physiological anticoagulants - antithrombin, proteins C and S (Andersson, 1997; Biron et al., 1997; Chan & Dixon, 2008; Curvers et al., 2001b; Nelson, 2009). Relationship between the predisposition to intravascular coagulation (thrombophilia) and unsuccessful ART results is actively discussed in current publications; however, mechanisms to produce the impact that increases thrombotic readiness on IVF are not absolutely clear. It is reported that women with thrombophilia may have increased risks for spontaneous abortion, preclinical pregnancy loss and recurrent implantation failure (Christiansen et al., 2006; Coulam et al., 2006b; Curnow et al., 2006; Many et al., 2001; Seghatchian et al., 1996; Stern & Chamley, 2006; Urman et al., 2005; Wichers et al., 2009; Younis et al., 2000). Presently, most studied and prevalent thrombophilias include APS and such risk factors as hereditary antithrombin III deficiency, factor V Leiden mutation, prothrombin mutation, polymorphism of methylenetetrahydrofolate reductase (MTHFR) gene, plasminogen activator inhibitor-1 (PAI-1), fibrinogen, platelet glycoproteins ITGA2, ITGB3, and some others. Beer and Kwak (2000) treated unsuccessful IVF programs as the evident indication for assays capable of detecting hereditary and acquired thrombophilias. In 2004, Azem et al. (2004) demonstrated higher occurrence of hereditary thrombophilia in women with multiple IVF failures as compared to the group of fertile women who became pregnant after the first IVF cycle. In the research conducted by Qublan et al. (2006), 69% of women with recurrent IVF failures had at least one hereditary or acquired thrombogenic risk factor as compared to 25% of women in the group where this reproductive technology was successful. In the publication presented by Grandone et al. (2001), factor V Leiden mutation prevailed (14.4%) in women with recurrent IVF failures as compared to the controls (1%). Recently, Coulam and Jeyendran (2009b) have shown that frequency of genetic polymorphisms has been 1.6 times higher in infertile women with IVF failures as compared to the fertile group; thus, polymorphism of the MTHFR gene has prevailed. It has been also noted that the connection of thrombogenic risk factors with recurrent miscarriages and repeated implantation failures after IVF is mainly evident in the simultaneous carriage of several thrombogenic mutations and polymorphisms (Coulam et al., 2006b).

Mechanisms of hemostasis and implantation pathologies typical of some thrombophilias (carriage of thrombogenic risk factors):

- factor V Leiden mutation (1691G>A). As long as activated protein C (APC) blocks activated factor V in regular conditions, resistance of the latter to APC can cause the increase of thrombinemia (Bertina et al., 1994; Dahlbäck et al., 1993). It is considered that patients who experience this mutation have higher risks for thrombosis and subsequent pregnancy loss. (Ridker et al., 1998; Urman et al., 2005; Younis et al., 2000);
- prothrombin mutation (20210G>A). This mutation is accompanied by the increased synthesis of prothrombin in the liver and increased risk for venous thrombosis (Girolami & Vianello, 2000; Poort et al., 1996);
- MTHFR gene polymorphism (C677>T) potentially causes increase in the level of homocysteine in blood (> 15 μmole/l), which affects human reproductive function (Nelen et al., 1998). In their publication Berker et al. (2009), interconnection between high level of homocysteine in the follicular fluid and decreased quality of oocytes and embryos in IVF programs has been discovered. High level of homocysteine in blood plasma relates to the decreased diameter of blood vessels located in the chorionic villi and miscarriage (Jerzak et al., 2003; Nelenet al., 2000). Thrombogenic action of homocysteine is based on the damage of endothelial cells, inhibition of prostacyclin synthesis, and increased platelet aggregation;
- PAI-1 gene polymorphism (5G>4G; 4G/4G) is related to the increased expression of PAI-1 in the blood plasma and endometrium, which disturbs the reaction of plasminogen activation into plasmin (Anteby et al., 2004; Buchholz et al., 2003; Ebish IM, et al., 2008; Kim et al., 1997);
- antiphospholipid syndrome. Damaging effect of antiphospholipid antibodies (APLAs) on oocytes and embryos on the early development stages has been indicated (Matsubayashi et al., 2006). Women with APS demonstrate high level of NK cells in the peripheral blood and endometrium. It is possible that disturbed synthesis of mediator molecules which participate in embryo adhesion and invasion by NK cells is one of the causes of disturbed signaling interaction between the blastocyst and endometrium on the earliest implantation stages (Quenby et al., 2009; Sher et al., 2000). APLAs stimulate PAI-1 synthesis that may cause disturbed degradation of intercellular matrix and decreased depth of blastocyst invasion.

Thus, making a brief summary, different forms of thrombophilia refer to different pathogenesis of implantation failures. Fixed and common conception for all thrombophilias is that pathology mechanisms are revealed in the earliest stages of pregnancy and are caused due to microcirculation and hemostasis disorders, as well as vessel wall pathology. Some researchers deny the impact of mutations of certain genes within the hemostasis system or isolated asymptomatic increase in the level of phospholipid antibodies on implantation. However, combination of several factors is believed to considerably increase individual risk of possible implantation failures and miscarriage. While estimating the occurrence of APS and mutations of genes participating in the hemostasis system in infertile women and women with IVF failures, specialists actively investigate qualitative changes on the level of endometrial structures and vascular endothelium accompanied by thrompophilia (Anteby et al., 2004; Coulam & Roussev, 2009a). Local mechanisms in the basis for implantation failures which occur along with thrombophilias are under investigated. Excessive activation of coagulation, imbalance in the coagulation system, endotheliopathy, local haemorrhages and microthrombi in the area of blastocyst invasion are common elements in the mechanism of implantation failures caused by thrombophilias. Thus, different forms of thrombophilia result in disorders on different stages of the coagulation cascade and fibrinolysis.

Analysis of publications demonstrates diverse expert opinions on the role of some mutations, polymorphisms of genes which are part of the hemostasis system and APS role in the development of infertility and ART failures. The American Society of Reproductive Medcine does not find it necessary to examine women who participate in IVF programs in order to detect risk factors for thrombophilia (American Society of Reproductive Medcine .., 2008). On the contrary, approach of the American Society for Reproductive Immunology to treat the same problem is completely opposite (American Society for Reproductive Immunology Antiphospholipid Antibody Committee .., 2000; Gleicher et al., 2002). Inconsistency of the opinions mentioned above may be explained by the absence of vast multicentral studies, use of diverse methodological approaches to diagnosing hemostasis pathologies and interpretation of examination results.

We believe that the most perspective approach in this area may be found in simultaneous consideration of thrombogenic risk factors and monitoring of the results collected with "global" methods which are capable of detecting disorders in the natural balance of pro- and anticoadulants in blood plasma under controlled ovarian hyperstimulation. This approach offers specialists the potential for the thrombin generation assay (TGA). This assay is known to define the dynamics and intensity of thrombin development; thrombin is the key hemostatic enzyme and relates to the group of integral indexes of the coagulation system (Hemker et al., 2000; Hemker et al., 2003; Hemker et al., 2006; Regnault et al., 2003; Wielders et al., 1997). This methodological approach has been successfully tested as a part of the complex estimation of the hemostasis system during pregnancy (Dargaud et al., 2010), preeclampsia (Macey et al., 2010) and oral contraceptive intake (Tchaikovski et al., 2007). Recent publication presented interesting data on the specifics of thrombin generation in blood plasma within IVF cycle (Westerlund et al., 2012). Shifts detected in 31 women were interpreted as the result of estrogen load and ovarian hyperstimulation syndrome and estimated to be vital for thrombosis prediction and IVF monitoring.

Besides, a number of researchers raise a great interest in the decrease of fibrinolytic blood activity, which is often detected in recurrent miscarriages, APS, deep vein thrombosis of lower extremities, oral contraceptive intake, myocardial infarction, and malignant neoplasms (Bertina, 1997; Birkenfeld et al., 1994; Curnow et al., 2006; Dmowski et al., 1995; Egbase et al., 1999; Lisman et al., 2005; Meltzer et al., 2009; Meltzer et al., 2010; Triplett, 1989; Wichers et al., 2009). The system of fibrinolysis, as well as the system of coagulation, is a complex system which gives characteristics to fibrinolytic responses and its central element that plays role in the activation of plasminogen into plasmin. Lately, its pathologies have been treated as new approach that explains the mechanisms of thrombosis pathogenesis (Zorio et al., 2008). The analysis of the fibrinolysis system during the IVF procedure shows the decrease in fibrinolytic responses due to several reasons (Andersson et al., 1997; Aune et al., 1991; Kim et al., 1981; Many et al., 2001; Martinez-Zamora et al., 2011; Meltzer et al., 2010; Nelson, 2009; Rice et al., 1993; Sarto et al., 2000). One of them is a decreased activity of tissue plasminogen activator (t-PA), increased level of its inhibitor - plasminogen activator inhibitor-1 (PAI-1), and increased level of thrombin-activatable fibrinolysis inhibitor (TAFI) dependent on the response of vascular endothelium (Bouma & Meijers, 2003; Martınez-Zamora et al., 2010; Martinez-Zamora et al., 2011; Meltzer et al., 2010).

4. Potential methods for the correction of hemostasis and fibrinolysis pathologies within the IVF program

Analysis of publications shows that correction of imbalanced homeostatic and fibrinolytic responses may be used in case of hormonal load within the IVF program accompanied by thrombophiia or present thrombogenic risk factors in a patient (Martinez-Zamora et al., 2011; Nelson & Greer, 2008; Rova et al., 2012; Urman et al., 2005). This is reasonable to determine thrombotic readiness, which becomes evident through the increase of general coagulation activity and thrombinemia and/or fibrinolysis suppression identified, for example, with the help of the thrombin generation assay upon detecting markers of thrombinemia and estimating fibrin clot lysis time for the fibrin obtained from euglobulins (Lisman et al., 2005; Wichers et al., 2009).

The use of heparins may become one of the methodologies aimed at the decrease of thrombogenicity and increase of IVF efficacy (Nelson & Greer, 2008; Urman et al., 2009). Still, there are no clear indications for the selection of women that need heparin prophylaxis within the IVF cycle.

Correction of hypofibrinolysis within IVF cycle also offers some difficulties for there are no published evidence of any successful drug therapy. Moreover, the hypothetic possibility to use pharmaceutical drugs - fibrinolysis activators (streptokinase, urokinase, and tissue plasminogen activator) - cannot be considered due to the absence of acute thrombosis. In the study conducted by Bjornsson et al. (1989), regular intake of aspirin in high doses (650 mg every 12 hours) caused the acceleration of fibrinolysis. But the mechanism of this effect is not absolutely clear, whereas the use of acetylsalicylic acid in high doses is unsafe due to the potential ulcerogenic effect. Nevertheless, it has been known for about 50 years that some stimuli (venous occlusion, physical load, desmopressin) lead to the acceleration of fibrinolytic responses facilitated by the fast increase of t-PA in blood due to its enhanced secretion by vascular endothelium. The effects of intermittent pneumatic compression (IPC) used to decrease the occurrence of postoperative venous thrombosis became our interests(Browse et al., 1977; Jacobs et al., 1996; Januszko et al., 1967; Holemans, 1963; Keber et al., 1979; Tarnay et al., 1980; Turpie et al., 1977; Weitz et al., 1986). Macdonald et al. (2003) published the results of their randomized pilot study demonstrating the efficacy of heparin prophylaxis combined with IPC in the course of neurosurgical invasions. The study conducted by Tarney et al. (1980) showed that intermittent compression of the calf, along with the increase in linear blood velocity and the decrease in venous stasis, increases local and systemic fibrinolytic potential (according to the shortened fibrin clot lysis time) in patients with acute myocardial infarction and prolonged movement disorders. Thus, the larger the volume of the compressed tissue gets, the more apparent became the response. The increase in blood and t-PA fibrinolytic activity after mechanical exposure on blood vessels is supported by the results presented by many authors (Bjornsson et al., 1989; Christen et al., 1997; Jacobs et al., 1996; Pandolfi et al.,1968; Salzman et al., 1987; Tarnay et al., 1980). However, we were not able to find any published data on the dynamics of PAI-1 activity. In the meantime, the correlation of the activities presented by these participants of the fibrinolysis system determines its overall efficacy. Some publications relate the mechanism of the IPC antithrombotic effect to the inhibition of coagulation cascade due to the expression of the tissue factor pathway inhibitor (TFPI) into blood flow and the decrease in the level of factor VIIa (Chouhan et al., 1999; Christen et al., 1997). Currently IPC is used worldwide for thromboprophylaxis in patients with strokes, after arthroplasty and a number of other operative invasions, in medical emergency,and applicable, firstly, in cases when administration of anticoagulants is dangerous due to the development of haemorrhage (Geerts & Selby, 2003; Gordon et al., 2012). As a rule, IPC is performed on the lower extremities, though some publications present positive results for the upper extremities compression (Knight & Dawson, 1976). Despite the fact that legs weigh more than arms, it was proved that forearm veins have considerably more t-PA than leg veins (Pandolfi et al., 1968). In our study this form of IPC was used to activate fibrinolytic responses within the IVF program and in the presence of relevant indications.

5. Original researches

This publication is based on the clinical study carried out to define the role of pathologies in the coagulation and fibrinolysis systems facilitating IVF failures, as well as to estimate the results of their correction.

In the framework of prospective analysis we collected data on 327 women who have been visiting the Center for Saving and Recovering the Reproductive Function, a subdivision of the Clinical Regional Hospital (Barnaul), from 2010 to 2012, to participate in the IVF program due to infertility. This study was approved by the Regional Ethics Committee of the Altai Medical University, and all the participants under study expressed their informed consent.

At the first visit women were interviewed about their obstetric, gynecological, and thrombotic history, possible diabetes, pathologies in the thyroid gland, heart and blood vessels. We have conducted ultrasonography of the genitals in order to detect organic pathologies of the pelvic organs and estimate the ovarian reserve (according to the quantity of antral follicles), aspiration biopsy and histologic examination of the endometrium, as well as to detect infections, including sexually transmitted diseases. We have also conducted general and special laboratory assays, including hormone panel assessment, blood chemistry panel, thrombogenic mutation and polymorphism carriage, coagulation profiles, and homocysteine presence. Then, based on the obtained results, women received professional consultation by obstetrician-gynecologists, physicians, and hematologists.

The study was chronologically conducted in two stages. At the first (observational) stage, we examined a random sampling of 163 women in their IVF cycle. At the second stage, we examined a random sampling of 164 women, 98 of which underwent the correction of the hemostasis and fibrinolysis systems in the presence of relevant indications - increased thrombin generation and/or decreased fibrinolytic activity of blood plasma (controlled group or group with the therapeutic effect on hemostasis and fibrinolysis) (Fig. 1).

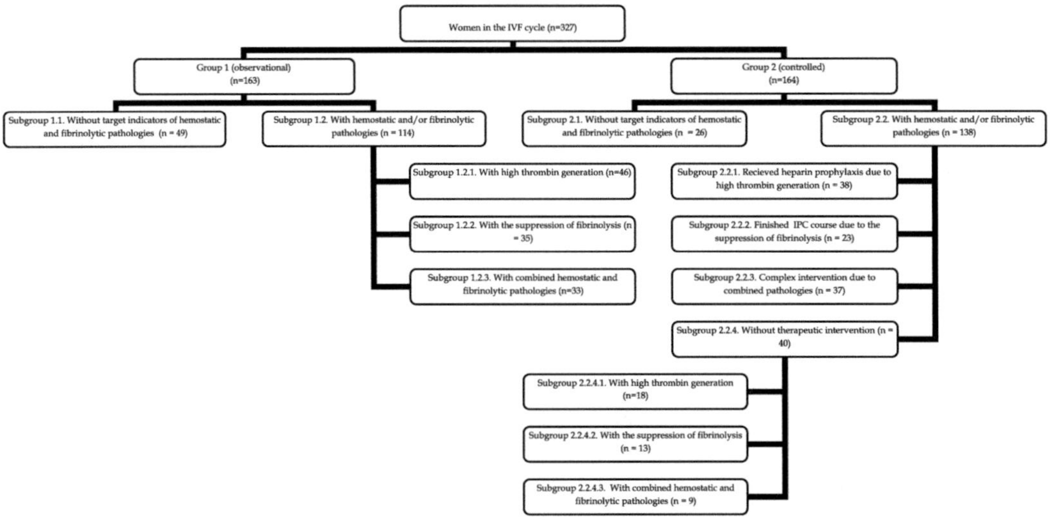

Figure 1. Division of women participating in the study into groups and subgroups

The selection criterion for the patients was any form of infertility non-responsive to traditional treatment. The exclusion criteria were somatic diseases serving as contraindications for carrying a pregnancy and delivery, congenital malformations or acquired deformations of the uterine cavity that make embryo implantation or carrying of a pregnancy impossible, ovarian tumors, benign uterine tumors that require operative invasion, malignant neoplasms.

All patients are representatives of the Caucasian race, their age ranged from 21 to 42 years (Table 1)

There was a difference in clinical profiles of women representing the two groups. The second group of patients suffers from chronic endometritis and has lower ovarian reserve. Besides, male infertility factor was more frequent in this group.

We used standard protocols to induce superovulation. In 72.4% (237 patients) of the whole population we used the "prolonged" protocol with diphereline (Ipsen) 0.1 mg or decapeptyl (Ferring) 0.1 mg and gonadotropic preparations - puregon (MSD) 150-250 IU, menopur (Ferring) 225 IU, or gonal (Merck Serono) 225 IU. In 27.6% (90 patients) of the whole population we stimulated superovulation using the same gonadotropic preparations and an antagonist - cetrotide (Merck Serono) 0.25 mg. Transvaginal follicle puncture was conducted with ultrosonic guidance using Medison Sonoace X8 machine. After we counted obtained oocytes and estimated their quality with the conventional scale (normal oocytes of good quality - 4-5 points, modified oocytes - less than 4 points), oocytes and embryos were cultivated in 6-well plates in the IVF medium (Vitrolife, Sweden), at 37 degrees Centigrade, in humid atmosphere containing 5% of CO2. Sperm processing was conducted with the Sil-Select Plus medium (FertiPro, Belgium). The ICSI procedure consisted of fertilization with the injection of a single sperm into the oocyte (177 married couples) in case of decreased sperm mobility or irregular sperm morphology. Embryo transfer was conducted with ultrasonic guidance on the 3rd day of cultivation. Embryos with the highest quality rating (A, AB) were selected for the transfer. Pregnancy was diagnosed two weeks after the embryo transfer by means of detecting b-human chorionic gonadotropin (b-hCG). After three weeks we defined quantity and location of the implanted embryos with ultrasonography (in 124 patients).

Indication	Total (n=327)	Group 1 (n=163)	Group 2 (n=164)	P-value*
Age, years (mean ± SD)	33.7 ± 4.1	33.2 ±3.6	34.4 ± 3.9	> 0.5
BMI > 25 kg/m², n (%)	61 (18.7)	34 (20.9)	27 (16.5)	0.323
Genital pathology:				
- Chronic endometritis, n (%)	**108 (33.0)**	**42 (25.8)**	**66 (40.2)**	**0.006**
- Endometriosis, n (%)	55 (16.8)	28 (17.2)	27 (16.5)	0.883
- Myoma, n (%)	45 (13.8)	25 (15.3)	20 (12.2)	0.426
IVF failure registered in the history, n (%)	36 (11.0)	19 (11.7)	17 (10.4)	0.727
Low ovarian reserve, n (%)	**55 (16.8)**	**19 (11.7)**	**36 (21.9)**	**0.017**
Extragenital pathology:				
- Hypothyroidism, n (%)	49 (15.0)	21 (12.9)	28 (17.1)	0.352
- Arterial hypertension, n (%)	6 (1.8)	2 (1.2)	4 (2.4)	0.684
Infertility causes:				
- Tubal factor, n (%)	119 (36.4)	61 (37.4)	58 (35.4)	0.730
- Male factor, n (%)	**138 (42.2)**	**59 (36.2)**	**79 (48.2)**	**0.033**
- Endocrinal factor, n (%)	29 (8.9)	14 (8.6)	16 (9.8)	0.848
Combination of female and male factors, n (%)	41 (12.5)	23 (14.1)	17 (10.7)	0.316

P-value* for within-group comparison (Fisher,s exact test); SD, standart deviation

Table 1. Clinical characteristic of the patients examined in the IVF cycle.

Technique of laboratory assays for hemostatic and fibrinolytic profiles.

Examination was conducted three times: 1-2 days before the start of controlled ovarian hyperstimulation and an IVF program (1st observation point), 2-3 days before the puncture of ovarian follicles (2nd observation point), and on the 12th-14th day after the embryo transfer (3rd observation point), when the outcome in terms of pregnancy was defined by estimating the level of b-hCG.

Sampling of venous blood was in the cubital vein in VACUETTE test tubes with the buffer solution of sodium citrate with the proportion of 9:1 (9NC Coagulation sodium citrate 3.2%). Blood was centrifuged at 1400 g and room temperature for 15 minutes. Plasma samples were generally studied within the two hours after being obtained. Prior to conducting immune-enzyme assays and estimating the endogenous thrombin potential, plasma was stored at -40 ^{degrees} Centigrade for the period of time ranging from 24 hours to 1 month.

Measuring of the endogenous thrombin potential was made as a part of the thrombin generation assay (TGA). We believe that this method may be regarded as a historical modification of the two-stage self-coagulogram suggested by Berkarda et al. (1965) and developed to pursue similar goals. It was demonstrated that TGA allows experts to measure the dynamics of thrombin generation and inactivation with high precision (Hemker et al., 2003; Hemker et al., 2006). To perform calibrated automated thrombography, the Fluoroskan Ascent microplate fluorometer was applied (Thermo Fisher Scientific, Finland) equiped with a dispenser with Thrombinoscope 3.0.0.26 software. Coagulation of plasma under study was conducted in the presence of tissue factor (5 μM) and phospholipids (4 μM); thrombin generation was continually registered by measuring the signal of fluorogenic substrate (Z-Gly-Gly-Arg-AMC). The following parameters were considered: endogenous thrombin potential (ETP, nM×min), calculating the area under the thrombin generation curve and taking into account specifics of the enzyme inactivation, and peak thrombin concentration - Peak thrombin (nM/l), maximal thrombin concentration per time unit.

Activity of t-PA and PAI-1 was defined by means of the immune-enzyme analysis with sets of reagents t-PA Combi Actibind ELISA Kit and Actibind PAI-1 ELISA (Technoclone, Austria), while the collected data was estimated by mutual comparison. Due to the fact that these important participants of fibrinolytic responses are antagonistic to each other and have a common origin (vascular endothelium), we calculated the index of endothelial ability to activate fibrinolysis (EAAF index). To do that we applied the following formula:

$$\text{EAAF index, \%} = \frac{\text{Activity of t} - \text{PA, un / ml}}{\text{Activity of PAI} - 1\text{, un / ml}} \times 100\%.$$

Defining clot lysis time (CLT). Many authors refer this method to the group of global assays for fibrinolysis assessment. It can be conducted in a variety of ways (Lisman et al., 2005; Martinez-Zamora et al., 2011; Wichers et al., 2009).

Method to define spontaneous lysis time of a fibrin clot obtained from plasma euglobulins was described by Kowarzyk and Buluk (1954). It is based on the precipitation of euglobulin fraction stabilized with sodium citrate in the acid medium with the simultaneous removal of fibrinolysis inhibitors. Then, following this methodology, specialists promote clot formation by recalcifying the reconstituted euglobulin solution and register period for its complete dissolution at fixed temperature (+37 ^{degrees} Centigrade). Martinez-Zamora et al. (2011) have recently published original CLT results obtained in women participating in IVF cycles using another method described by Lisman et al. (2002). In particular, this method implies the study of CLT for clots obtained from blood plasma by means of activitaing fibrinolysis with exogenous t-PA. For our study we use a modified method suggested by Kowarzyk and Buluk (1954) and used kaolin that activates the contact phase of coagulation and starts activation cascade. Factor XIIa →kallikrein →plasmin. Description of this method was given earlier by Barkagan and Momot [Barkagan Z.S., Momot A.P. Diagnosis and controlled therapy of hemostasis pathologies. / M., Publisher: Nyudiamed-AO, 2001. - 296 P.]. Range of normal CLT variations in this modification is 8-12 minutes.

Definition of the D-dimer concentration in blood plasma was conducted with the help of reagent set D-dimer Red-700 (Helena Bioscience, UK) and blood coagulation analyzer Sysmex CA-1500 (Sysmex, Japan). This parameter was considered in accordance with conventional conceptions as a global marker for the completion of fibrin generation and fibrinolysis of stabilized fibrin.

Definition of gene mutations and polymorphisms, predisposing to thrombosis, was conducted with the method of polymerase chain reaction. Thus, we detected the carriers of factor V Leiden (1691G>A) and factor II (20210G>A) mutations, MTHFR (C677>T) and PAI-1 gene polymorphisms related to potential activation of coagulation or decreased plasmin generation, as well as to IVF failures and miscarriages (Coulam et al., 2006a).

5.1. Statistical analysis

Statistical processing of the obtained data was made with the following software: Microsoft Office Excel 2003, Statistica 6.1, and Medcalc 12.2.1. Validity of the differences in mean values was defined with the Student's t-test (t). Group distribution normalcy was estimated with the Shapiro-Wilk test. In cases when the distribution deviated from the norm, we used the non-parametric Mann-Whitney U test for two independent groups and the Spearman's rank correlation coefficient (R). For experimental data presented in percentages or rates the Fisher's exact test was used. Odds ratio (OR) and log-linear rate analysis were calculated as a measure of predictor impact. To estimate the accuracy of obtained values, we defined a 95% confidence interval. Differences $P<0.05$ were considered statistically significant. We assessed the efficacy of the chosen treatment methods with conventional criteria applied in evidence-based medicine, including Absolute Risk Reduction (ARR), Relative Risk (RR), Relative Risk Reduction (RRR), Number Needed to Treat (NNT), and Confidence Interval (CI).

5.2. Study results

5.2.1. Estimation of hemostatic and fibrinolytic indications in the IVF cycle and definition of threshold values occurring in the assay results for the selection of women who need therapeutic intervention during the controlled ovarian hyperstimulation

At the beginning of the study, it was important to investigate shifts in the hemostatic and fibrinolytic systems that may affect IVF outcomes (in terms of the pregnancy rate) and to define their quantitative level that may help in selecting those women who need the correction of disturbed hemostatic and fibrinolytic responses. As a result, we defined that thrombin generation in the observational group had considerably increased after the start of controlled ovarian hyperstimulation in response to a sharp increase in the level of estrogens in blood, which is consistent with recently published data (Westerlund et al., 2012). We have also found that the degree of the increase in thrombin generation is different at successful and unsuccessful IVF outcomes (Table 2). In particular, the values of such thrombin generation factors as ETP and peak thrombin concentration at the 2nd observation point were higher in case of IVF failures (P<0.001) as compared with the similar data in patients with pregnancies.

Indication	At IVF failure (n=107)			At pregnancy (n=56)		
	1st observation point	2nd observation point	3rd observation point	1st observation point	2nd observation point	3rd observation point
ETP, nM/min	1655±39.2**	2060.5±52.7**	1853.9±55.6**	1574.8±36.9	1723±54.2	1632.7±56.4
Peak thrombin concentration, nM/l	328.6±24.8**	394.1±25.6**	378.4±25.5**	313.2±24.6	338.3±25.5	310.1±26.0
t-PA, activity, un/ml	0.36±0.16	0.37±0.18	0.38±0.18	0.37±0.14	0.36±0.16	0.35±0.17
PAI-1, activity, un/ml	4.22±2.98	4.08±2.76	4.10±2.16	3.67±2.68	3.41±2.87	3.25±2.31
EAAF index, %	8.5±3.4	9.1±4.1	9.3±4.2	10.0±4.1	10.5±4.9	10.7±4.6
Clot lysis time, min	13.5±3.7*	14.3±3.9*	14.9±3.8*	11.2±3.5	11.9±2.9	12.5±3.3
D-dimers, ng/ml	223.7±31.7**	266.4±27.8*	321.0±31.4**	198.5±25.4	251.6±26.1	298.4±28.4

t – test; * - in this table, as well as in tables 5, 8-11, the validity of differences P<0.05 between the groups characterized by different outcomes occurring within the same observation periods of the IVF cycle; ** - the same, P<0.01.

Table 2. Quantitative level and change dynamics of hemostatic and fibrinolytic indications (mean ± SD) in women of the 1st (observational) group (n=163)

The most significant adverse indication for this reproductive technology was ETP value, which range limits at different IVF outcomes in the middle of the cycle did not intersect even with the M ± 3SD limit (Fig. 2). Peack thrombin concentration also changed, but its values in the compared groups did not intersect within the M ± SD limit.

With regard to the conducted studies, the threshold value for the positive decision on administering heparin prophylaxis was set according to the following criteria: ETP exceeds 1900 nM/min and/or increased Peack thrombin concentration of over 360 nM/l.

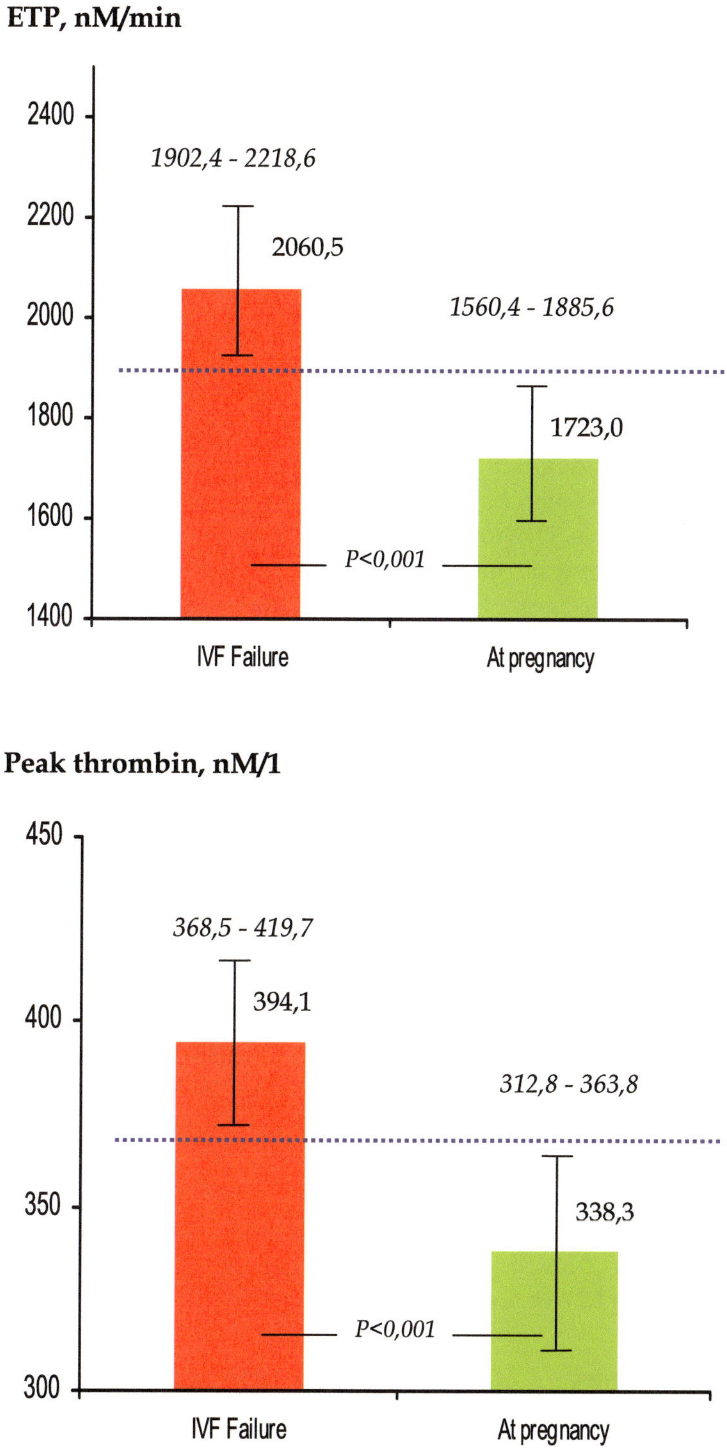

Figure 2. Definition of the threshold values for TGA indications (ETP and peak thrombin concentration) at different IVF outcomes in the 1st (observational) group (at the 2nd observation point).

The level of D-dimers, a known marker for fibrin generation and fibrinolysis, showed less distinctive differences in subgroups 1.1 and 1.2, even though it was slightly decreased, according to the mean data, in case of IVF failures (Table 2). Mean values of this indication in virtually healthy women of fertile age registered in our Center were equal to 205.3 ng/ml, with M ± 2SD 148.5 - 262.1 ng/ml. Respectively, registered results of the D-dimer level at the 2nd observation point were within the allowed value limits or slightly exceeded them.

It was more difficult to define the threshold values that reflect the decrease in the activity of fibrinolytic responses and allow specialists to select patients in need of hypofibrinolysis correction. Recent important publications devoted to this field demonstrate that hypofibrinolysis may be typical of some women who participate in the IVF procedure, but this pathology is original and not triggered in the course of controlled hormonal stimulation as a part of the IVF program (Martinez-Zamora et al., 2011; Westerlund et al. 2012). We received similar data proving that the suppression of fibrinolytic responses was actually typical of a number of women before the beginning of the IVF cycle. Suppression was steady throughout the cycle. Dynamics analysis of the changes in t-PA and PAI-1 activities, their EAAF index, and clot lysis time revealed more dramatic shifts at IVF failures, though the difference between the mean values of the parameters under study turned out to be invalid (P<0.05) (Table 2). Nevertheless, we have recorded two facts. First, mean values of the EAAF index defined in the group of 10 virtually healthy female volunteers (20-23 years) were equal (M±SD) to 11.0±3.3%. Second, in case of IVF failures we registered decreased EAAF indexes (less than 11%) in 93.5% (43 out of 46) of women in the 1st (observational) group before the start of the IVF program (1st observational point) as compared to 4,1% (2 out of 49) of women after successful impregnation (P<0.000001) (Table 3).

We used the values of the applied CLT assay to be the method of general fibrinolysis monitoring and refused to consider it as a potential criterion for the selection of women in need of therapeutic invasion in relation to its laboratory standardization. Thus, to select females to undergo IPC procedure we chose EAAF index calculation rate, which records the correlation between t-PA and PAI-1 activities, with the value of less than 11%.

Back to the data presented above and obtained during the study of the hemostasis and fibrinolysis systems in the patients of the 1st or observational group (n=163), one can see significant correlation between the detected pathologies and certain IVF outcomes (Table 3). Adverse shifts in these systems had records in 114 out of 163 women (70%) in the 1st group. In general, the IVF cycle efficacy at this stage of the study was equal to 34.4%, however, certain hemostatic and fibrinolytic pathologies facilitated the decrease in the number of successful impregnations from 95.9% (47 out of 49 women in subgroup 1.1) to 7.9% (9 out of 114 women in subgroup 1.2), i.e. in 12.1 times (P<0,000001).

5.2.2. Results of the therapeutic invasion in the hemostatic and fibrinolytic systems administered for the increase in the number of successful IVF outcomes

Correction of the hemostatic system at the excessive thrombin generation initially arranged the administration of heparin prophylaxis by means of subcutaneous introduction of nadroparin calcium (Sanofi-Aventis): 0.3 ml twice a day for 12-14 days. Decision to begin the therapy was based on marking a suprathreshold increase in the major indications of thrombin generation - ETP (over 1900 nM/min) and/or Peack thrombin concentration (over 360 nM/l) at the 2nd observation point.

Patient subgroups	Abs. (n=163)	% of the whole study populatio n	Impregnation	
			Abs. (n=56)	% of pregnant women
1.1. Without target indicators of hemostatic and fibrinolytic pathologies	49	30.1	47	83.9
1.2. With hemostatic and fibrinolytic pathologies	114	69.9	9	16.1
1.2.1. With ETP exceeding 1900 nM/min and/or increased Peack thrombin concentration of over 360 nM/l (at the 2nd observational point)	46	28.2	3	5.4
1.2.2. With decreased EAAF index of less than 11% and prolonged clot lysis time of over 12 min. (at the 1st observational point)	35	21.5	4	7.1
1.2.3. With ETP exceeding 1900 nM/min and/or increased Peack thrombin concentration of over 360 nM/l (at the 2nd observational point) and decreased EAAF index of less than 11% (at the 1st observational point)	33	20.2	2	3.6

Table 3. IVF results in women of the 1st (observational) group depending on the presence or absence of hemostatic and fibrinolytic pathologies

Impact on the vessel wall to increase fibrinolytic activity was made by means of IPC. In the publication byKakkos et al. (2005) a comparative description of the two widely used compression machines - SCD Express™ Compression System (Tyco Healthcare Group LP, Mansfield, MA, USA) was introduced with a rapid inflation device that delivers uniform compression and VenaFlow® (Aircast Inc, Summit, NJ, USA). However neither of them is normally equipped with proper braces to provide mechanical invasion for arm vessels. Still, we found it important to compress this vessel area to exclude even the hypothetic possibilty

Subgroups examined	Abs. (n=164)	% of total number of women	Impregnation	
			Abs. (n=68)	% of number of pregnant
2.1. Without the required signs of pathology of hemostasis and fibrinolysis	26	15,8	21	30,9
2.2. Without the required signs of pathology of hemostasis and fibrinolysis	138	84,2	47	69,1
- including an increase in ETP over 1900 nM/min and/or with Peack thrombin more than 360 nM/l (2nd point of observation)	50	30,5	19	27,9
- including those with reduced EAAF index less than 11% (on the 1st point of observation)	40	24,4	14	20,6
- including an increase in ETP over 1900 nM/min and/or increased Peack thrombin more than 360 nM/l (2nd point of observation) and a decrease of the index EAAF less than 11% (on the 1st point of observation)	48	29,3	14	20,6
Received treatment against diseases of hemostasis, including:	98	59,8	42	61,8
2.2.1. After heparin prophylaxis	38	23,2	15	22,1
2.2.2. After IPC course	23	14,0	10	14,7
2.2.3. When combined IPC course with heparin prophylaxis	37	22,6	17	25
2.2.4. Those in need of treatment, but did not receive it	40	24,4	5	7,3

Table 4. Results of IVF in women of the 2nd (controlled) group in relation to the presence or absence of disorders in hemostasis and fibrinolysis

of the pulmonary artery thromboembolia (e.g. in the presence of clinically non-evident iliofemoral thrombosis) and due to the obtained data on the increased content of t-Pa in endotelial vessels of the upper extremities (Pandolfi et al., 1968). That is why we chose pneumatic massaging device PM-01 (Russia) to apply a 7-chamber compression brace in the upper arm area using the mode of wave compression with the following parameters:

chambers from 30 to 150 mm. Hg. Art., 45 cycles of compression wave with memory for 30 minutes to maintain the pressure in the cuff chambers from 5 to 90., the pressure of compressed air supplied to the compression performed in a course of 8 sessions (twice a week) with 30-minute cuff device to the left or right hand. The starting point of this therapy was to reduce EAAF index below 11% measured in a number of patients just prior to IVF program (1st point of observation).

Studies have found that the total number of favorable outcomes of IVF in the 2nd (controlled) group was 41.5%, an increase of only 7.1%, compared with those in group 1 (34.4%; P <0,21) (Table 3 and Table 4).

However, please note that 40 patients (subgroup 2.2.4) failed our proposed therapy, although prescribed by the above criteria. If to sum up the outcome of IVF in all samples in the study of women who had indications for treatment but did not receive it for a number of reasons (sub 1.2 and 2.2.4; 154 cases) we indicate positive results in 9.1%, whereas in the treated patients (subgroup 2.2.1, 2.2.2 and 2.2.3, 98 cases) - in 42.9%, or 4.71 times more likely (P<0,000001).

Effect of treatment produced on the dynamics of hemostasis and fibrinolysis during IVF is shown in Table 5. You can see the previous trends in Table 2, but the women in group 2, compared to the 1 st group demonstrated lower intensity of thrombin generation and improvement of fibrinolysis regardless of the outcome of IVF.

D-dimer levels in blood plasma has indicated growing trend - the concentration of this indicator has been consistently higher regardless of the period of the survey in patients with unsuccessful IVF outcome (Tables 2 and 5). However, the value of D-dimer levels was within the range of normal variation or slightly exceeded them, hardly matching the identified changes parameters under study (Table 6).

In this regard, we have not put the emphasis on the results of this test upon the following analysis.

Other risk factors of unsuccessful IVF which did not depend on the characteristics of hemostatic and fibrinolytic had its effect on IVF success (see Section 2, Table 13, 14), as well as the fact of receiving or not receiving therapeutic intervention aimed at reducing the thrombogenic potential and increasing fibrinolytic activity of blood. Calculations and observations in tables 7-12 demonstrate a better pattern in this regard. In particular, it appeared that an approved prescription of low-molecular heparin at high thrombin generation at the 2nd stage of the study contributed to the increase in the incidence of pregnancy in 6.4 times (P<0,0001), isolated IPC course application -in 3.0 times (P<0,007), and the combination of IPC course with heparin prophylaxis - in 6.5-times (P<0,0001) (Table 7).

Indication	At failure in IVF cycle (n=96)			At pregnancy (n=68)		
	First point of observation	Second point of observation	Third point of observation	First point of observation	Second point of observation	Third point of observation
ETP, nM/min	1825,3±96,8*	1922,1±64,7*	1785,4±±89,5	1645,6±54,9	1762,1±79,8	1711,2±84,3
Peack thrombin, nM/l	342,1±26,3**	381,5±25,7**	364,4±24,3**	310,7±27,4	329,1±29,3	326,4±25,7
t-PA, activity un/ml	0,35±0,14	0,51±0,15	0,48±0,13	0,35±0,15	0,47±0,16	0,44±0,14
PAI-1, activity un/ml	3,55±1,75	2,64±1,91	2,32±1,58	3,48±2,11	1,95±0,75	1,86±0,57
EAAF index, %	9,9±4,28	19,3±3,88*	20,6±4,53*	10,0±3,97	24,1±4,39	23,6±4,77
Clot lysis time, min	15,5±3,65	12,3±3,86	11,4±4,04	13,4±3,85	11,8±3,85	10,1±3,11
D-dimers, ng/ml	236,4±26,2*	258,6±25,1*	305,6±28,5*	194,7±32,4	233,4±24,5	211,7±28,6

Table 5. The dynamics of hemostasis and fibrinolysis (M ± SD) in women of second (controlled) group (n = 164), t - test

Indication	Rank correlation	P value
ETP, nM/min	0,09	0,017
Peack thrombin, nM/l	0,125	0,002
t-PA, activity, un/ml	0,118	0,0003
PAI-1, activity, un/ml	0,124	0,0004
EAAF index, %	0,107	0,0006
Clot lysis time, min	0,111	0,0005

Table 6. Pair correlation between the level of D-dimers (by Spearman) and the study of hemostasis and fibrinolysis in different periods of the IVF cycle, regardless of its outcome

Modality	In need of treatment, but did not receive it (sub-1.2 and 2.2.4; n = 154)			In need of treatment, and treated (sub 2.2.1, 2.2.2 and 2.2.3; n = 98)		
	Abs.	Became pregnant	%	Abs.	Became pregnant	%
1. Heparin Prophylaxis	64	4	6,2	38	15	39,5
2. IPC course	48	7	14,6	23	10	43,5
3. Combined effect	42	3	7,1	37	17	45,9

Table 7. The influence of the methods of correction of hemostatic and fibrinolytic responses to the effectiveness of IVF (with data 1 and 2 stage of the research)

Criteria such as Absolute Risk Reduction (ARR), Relative Risk (RR), Relative Risk Reduction (RRR), Number Needed to Treat (NNT), Confidence Interval (CI) were determined for further evaluation of the effectiveness of the treatment (Table 8).

Modality	Indication					
	ARR	NNT	OR	CI 95% (RRR)	CI 95% (OR)	RRR%
Heparin Prophylaxis	0,27	3,7	0,22	0,52-0,92	0,07-0,69	31
IPC Course	0,31	3,2	0,19	0,44-0,94	0,05-0,65	35
Heparin prophylaxis combined with IPC course	0,55	1,8	0,24	0,23-0,60	0,02-0,22	63

Table 8. The effectiveness of different methods of therapy in women in a cycle of IVF

Indication	In need of treatment, but did not receive it (subgroup 1.2 и 2.2.4; n=154)			In need of treatment, and treated (subgroup 2.2.1, 2.2.2 и 2.2.3; n=98)		
	First point of observation	Second point of observation	Third point of observation	First point of observation	Second point of observation	Third point of observation
ETP, nM/min	1459,4±85,1	1912,5±108,6**	1872,8±85,1**	1490,6±84,1	1729,8±89,5	1566,4±72,7
Peack thrombin, nM/l	307,1±31,8	391,2±25,3**	385,4±22,5**	313,1±19,7	362,8±23,1	341,3±25,6
t-PA, activity, un/ml	0,32±0,15	0,34±0,16	0,33±0,15	0,34±0,12	0,48±0,15	0,49±0,14
PAI-1, activity, un/ml	3,18±2,32	3,22±1,66	3,26±1,75	3,22±1,71	2,76±1,51	2,68±1,67
EAAF index, %	10,0±3,2	10,5±4,3**	10,1±4,1**	10,5±3,5	17,3±4,4	18,2±4,2
Clot lysis time, min	13,1±3,6	14,2±3,9	15,4±3,8**	12,2+4,4	10,1±4,5	9,2±3,4

Table 9. The dynamics of hemostasis and fibrinolysis (M ± SD) in women in a cycle of IVF when indicated for the correction of hemostasis (n = 138), t - test

The choice was made towards absence of pregnancy after conducted treatment as the negative outcome of IVF. The control group included 154 women who had revealed violations of blood coagulation and fibrinolysis and did not receive treatment (subgroups 1.2 and 2.2.4). The intervention group had patients who received one of three therapies aimed at correcting identified violations in the hemostatic system and hypofibrinolysis (subgroup 2.2.1, 2.2.2, 2.2.3). It was discovered that all of the treatment reduced the risk of a negative outcome of IVF. In particular, in order to prevent one adverse outcome, you need to treat 2 women by the combined treatment option (1.8), using the IPC - 3 women (3.2), and heparin prophylaxis - 4 women (3.7). The relative risk reduction (RRR) in all cases was greater than 25%, which corresponded to clinical effect, and upon combined RRR therapy more than 50%, indicated a pronounced clinical effect.

Evolution of indicators reflecting defects of hemostatic and fibrinolytic reactions in patients in need of therapeutic intervention are shown in Table 9. Obviously, undertaken treatment has a beneficial effect on the rate of thrombin generation and fibrinolysis, and the index EAAF which reflects fibrinolysis-activation ability of the vascular wall indicated the increase in 2 times.

We also made separate calculations of laboratory parameters in women with high thrombin generation in need of heparin prophylaxis (Table 10). As a result, it was found that low molecular weight heparin with a mid-cycle IVF significantly reduces the generation of thrombin. In particular, the background rate nadroparin ETP between the 2nd and 3rd observation points decreased by 18.1%, compared to 3.6% in women who did not receive anticoagulant. The similar dynamics had Peack thrombin, which decreased, respectively, by 13.2% and 1.8%.

Indication	In need of treatment, but did not receive it (subgroup 1.2.1. и 2.2.4.1; n=64)			At heparin prophylaxis (subgroup 2.2.1; n=38)		
	First point of observation	Second point of observation	Third point of observation	First point of observation	Second point of observation	Third point of observation
ETP, nM/min	1461,2±81,6	1849,3±89,2	1782,4±93,5**	1489,5±85,5	1861,2±94,4	1524,6±88,9
Peack thrombin, nM/l	310,1±23,1	382,4±19,5	375,6±25,2**	321,2±22,3	386,3±23,5	335,2±20,2
t-PA, activity, un/ml	0,30±0,16	0,33±0,15	0,31±0,15	0,33±0,12	0,41±0,16	0,42±0,17
PAI-1, activity, un/ml	2,40±1,13	2,50±1,22	2,44±1,98	2,84±1,45	3,61±1,75	3,50±1,71
EAAF index, %	12,5±3,1	13,2±4,2	12,7±3,6	11,62±3,2	11,35±4,2	12,0±3,9
Clot lysis time, min	9,4±3,0	8,7±3,3	10,1±3,5	8,4±3,7	8,7±2,8	9,7±3,2

Table 10. The dynamics of hemostasis and fibrinolysis (M ± SD) in the second group of women in the presence of indications for heparin prophylaxis (n = 102), t – test

It should be noted that the indicators of fibrinolytic activity has not changed and remained stable without regard to heparin and duration of the study.

Indication	In need of treatment, but did not receive it (subgroup 1.2.2. и 2.2.4.2; n=48)			IPC Course recipients (subgroup 2.2.2.2; n=23)		
	First point of observation	Second point of observation	Third point of observation	First point of observation	Second point of observation	Third point of observation
ETP, nM/min	1534,4±87,2**	1575,7±85,6	1589,6±96,4	1415,1±87,7	1562,3±86,1	1632,3±93,8
Peack thrombin, nM/l	314,2±30,3*	322,4±28,2	327,7±25,7**	294,5±24,4	322,1±31,1	353,3±25,9
t-PA, activity, un/ml	0,36±0,14	0,39±0,15	0,37±0,14*	0,35±0,16	0,51±0,15	0,48±0,15
PAI-1, activity, un/ml	3,98±1,67	4,11±2,32	4,05±2,54*	3,55±1,88	2,64±1,06	2,32±1,32
EAAF index, %	9,0±3,2	9,5±3,6**	9,1±4,0**	9,9±3,2	19,3±3,4	20,6±4,5
Clot lysis time, min	13,8±4,3	14,4±4,6*	14,8±3,2**	14,3±4,1	11,4±3,7	9,0±3,3

Table 11. The dynamics of hemostasis and fibrinolysis (M ± SD) in the second group of women in the event of Table readings for IPC course (n = 71), t – test

Indication	In need of treatment, but did not receive it (subgroup 1.2.3 и 2.2.4.3; n=42)			At heparin prophylaxis and IPC course recipients (subgroup 2.2.3; n=37)		
	First point of observation	Second point of observation	Third point of observation	First point of observation	Second point of observation	Third point of observation
ETP, nM/min	1538,6±78,3	1770,4±85,6	1756,6±95,7**	1566,7±86,3	1764,4±95,7	1542,1±81,3
Peack thrombin, nM/l	322,3±32,4	379,3±29,1	374,5±31,6**	324,7±27,6	371,2±33,8	335,6±30,7
t-PA, activity, un/ml	0,37±0,17	0,39±0,15	0,36±0,16	0,31±0,16	0,49±0,15	0,46±0,14
PAI-1, activity, un/ml	3,64±2,05	4,12±1,77	3,45±1,98	3,02±1,69	2,29±1,14	2,09±0,91
EAAF index, %	10,2±2,9	9,5±3,1**	10,4±3,3**	10,2±2,6	21,4±4,5	22,0±4,3
Clot lysis time, min	15,4±3,9	13,2±4,2**	15,7±3,4**	13,8±2,3	10,0±3,8	9,1±3,9

Table 12. The dynamics of hemostasis and fibrinolysis (M ± SD) in the second group of women when indicated for combination therapy (n = 79), t – test

Similar calculations were performed in women with hypofibrinolysis as well as with the combination of low fibrinolytic activity with excessive generation of thrombin (Tables 11 and 12). It was found that the isolated effects of IPC in women with original, prior to the IVF cycle hypofibrinolysis indicated a sharp increase in EAAF index combined with the decrease in CLT. Interestingly, vases compression led to the significant increase of t-PA activity as well as to the reduction of PAI-1activity at the end of the IVF cycle. It was also discovered that the application of IPC led to increased thrombin generation which Peack thrombin factor clearly demonstrated.

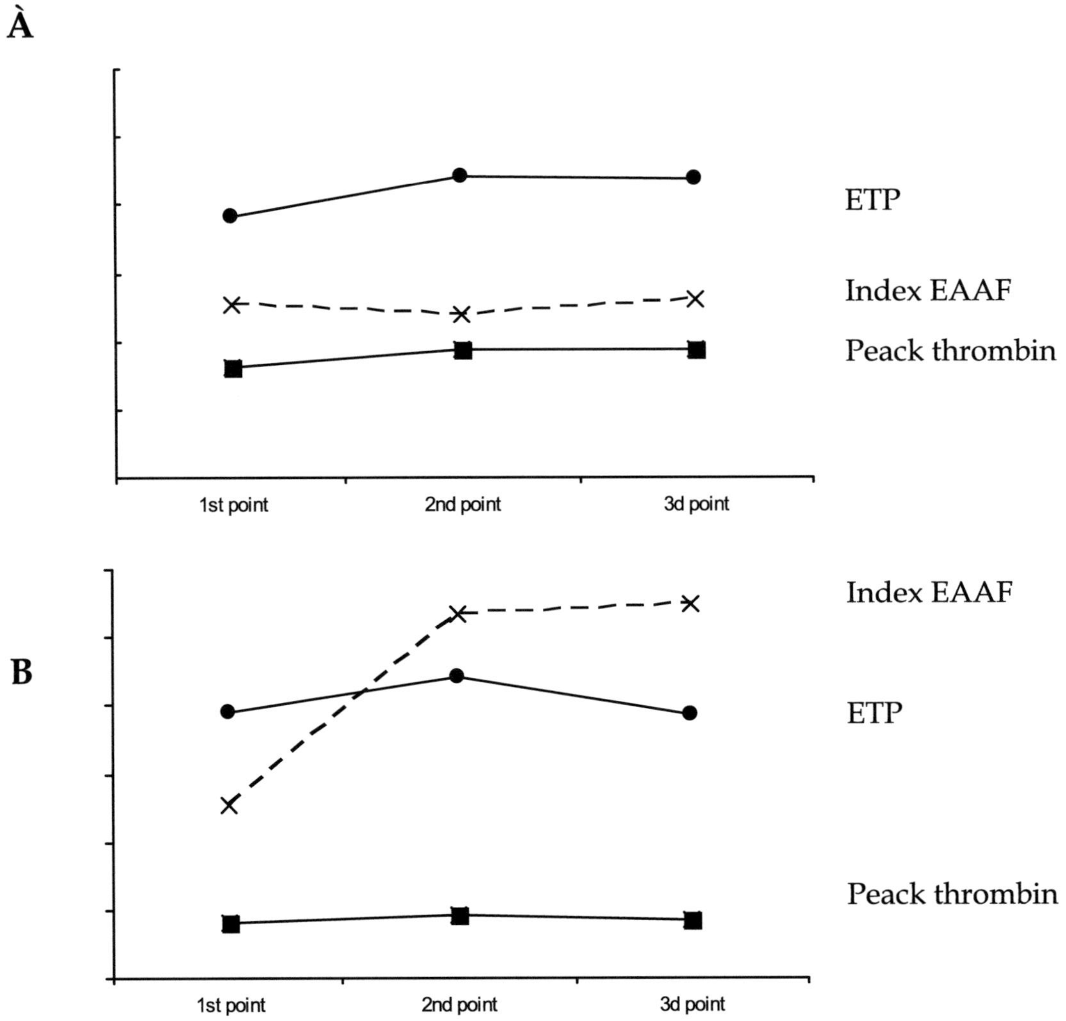

Figure 3. The evolution of laboratory parameters of hemostasis and fibrinolysis in women who require concomitant therapy, but do not receive it (A) during such therapy (B)

Combined application of IPC and low molecular weight heparin produced complex beneficial effect on hemostasis and fibrinolysis to be in correspondence with the maximum increase in the number of IVF successful outcomes (Tables 4, 7, 8 and 12).

In Fig. 3 the dynamics of the main parameters studied in the course of the treatment for the correction of hemostasis and fibrinolysis is highlighted.

5.2.3. Comparative analysis of the prognostic value of a number of factors contributing to the failure of IVF

This section has recorded and compared the effect of risk factors in the failure of IVF in 1st (observation) group and women of (2nd) group. We studied a wide range of adverse prognostic factors which are well-known in Reproduction and discussed in this publication: markers of thrombogenic risk and blood fibrinolytic activity reduction as well as hyperhomocysteinemia, thrombogenic mutations and polymorphisms carriers, presence of an inflammatory response (Bates et al., 2008; Coulam & Jeyendran, 2009b; Heit, 2007; Qublan & Eid, 2006), "0" blood type negative factor [Canonico et al., 2008; Ohira et al., 2007.)

Assessing the reasons for the failure of pregnancy in IVF cycles in 163 patients of the 1st (observation) group based on the analysis of the odds ratio (OR), 9 out of 27 (33.3%) factors became the most important adverse factors or symptoms to be rated as fairly significant (Table 13). Importantly, indicators reflecting increased thrombin generation and inhibition of fibrinolytic reactions, respectively, 2nd and 3d entered the adverse factors as well. Hypo fibrinolysis factors with high reliability proved to be at the 5th and 6th adverse factors ranking. Consequently, in addition to well-known factors listed in Section 2, increased ability to thrombosis, in response to the stress estrogen and inhibition of fibrinolytic reactions are among the leading causes of failure of IVF. It is interesting to note that such a well-known and widely used in clinical practice marker of thrombinemia as high D-dimer plasma levels did not vary in frequency of occurrence in impregnate women at all stages of observation (OR 0,99; 0,95% CI 0,42-2,31 – 21 rank).

Carriage of thrombogenic mutations and polymorphisms were identified in the majority of our patients (71.2%). By the rare mutations - Factor V Leiden and prothrombin in only 4 cases (2.4%), we cannot judge the significance of their influence. However, the combination of polymorphisms MTGFR and PAI-1 was found in a slightly larger percentage of cases with unsuccessful IVF (24.3% vs. 16.0%) to be, however, insignificant. Interestingly, blood type "not 0"did not prove to be protrombogen/unfavorable by nature in our observation as well as a number of variants of virus infection carriers and the manifestations of inflammation (fibrinosis, leukocytosis).

The number of factors contributing to the failure of pregnancy in IVF changed dramatically after exposure to therapeutic correction of hemostasis and fibrinolysis, used in the present publication. In accordance with the data in Table 14, traditional reasons for Reproduction are among the leaders: early hyperstimulation, male factor, and others. Hyperhomocysteinemia (OR 3,45; 0,95% CI 1,16-10,2) became one of the hemostatic reasons at the 4th rank to be the result of obvious lack of attention to the problem of metabolic methionine in preparation for IVF protocol. The significance level of manifestation of high thrombin generation shifted from the 2nd and 3rd rank to 8th and 9th rank whereas EAAF index - from 6th to 15th rank to be the further proof of the effectiveness of our methods of applied therapeutic intervention. Please, note that the calculations in this table exclude 40 patients with disorders of hemostasis and fibrinolysis who did not receive treatment for a number of reasons (subgroup 2.2.4).

Criterion	Failure of IVF (n=107)		Success of IVF (n=56)		Odds ratio (0,95% CI)	P-value
	Abs.	%	Abs.	%		
1. Hyperstimulation (early stage)	22	20,5	0	0	29,7 (1,76-500)	< 0,00001
2. ETP more than 1900 nM/min (2nd point of observation)	73	68,2	4	7,1	27,9 (9,33-83,4)	< 0,00001
3. Peack thrombin more than 360 nM/L (2nd point of observation)	74	69,1	5	8,9	22,8 (8,36-62,5)	< 0,00001
4. Oligozoospermia (moderate and severe)	45	42,0	2	3,5	19,5 (4,53-84,6)	< 0,00001
5. Clot lysis time of over 12 minutes (1st point of observation)	69	64,5	5	8,9	18,5 (6,81-50,3)	< 0,000001
6. EAAF index less than 11% (1st point of observation)	62	57,9	6	10,7	11,5 (4,53-29,1)	0,00005
7. Defective embryo	23	21,4	3	5,3	4,83 (1,38-16,9)	0,011
8. Insufficient number of embryos transferred in IVF cycles (1-2)	38	35,5	6	10,7	4,58 (1,80-11,6)	0,0007
9. Mutation FV (G/A, A/A)	3	2,8	0	0	3,78 (0,19-74,5)	0,319
10. Difficult embryo transfer	32	29,9	6	10,7	3,55 (1,38-9,12)	0,006
11. Hypoplasia of the endometrium	11	10,3	3	5,3	2,02 (0,54-7,57)	0,383
12. Unsuccessful IVF attempt in history	20	18,7	6	10,7	1,91 (0,72-5,08)	0,260
13. Homocysteine in blood of more than 15 mM/l (1st point of observation)	22	20,5	7	12,5	1,81 (0,72-4,54)	0,280
14. Age (36-40 years)	19	17,7	6	10,7	1,79 (0,67-4,80)	0,262

Criterion	Failure of IVF (n=107)		Success of IVF (n=56)		Odds ratio (0,95% CI)	P-value
	Abs.	%	Abs.	%		
15. High dose-protocol	35	32,7	12	21,4	1,78 (0,83-3,79)	0,148
16. The combination of polymorphisms MTHFR (C/T, T/T) and PAI-I (5 G/4 G, 4 G/4 G)	26	24,3	9	16,0	1,67 (0,72-3,87)	0,315
17. Low ovarian reserve	19	17,7	7	12,5	1,51 (0,59-3,84)	0,500
18. Polymorphism of PAI-I (5 G/4 G, 4 G/4 G)	42	39,2	20	35,7	1,16 (0,59-2,27)	0,735
19. Cytomegalovirus infection	11	10,3	5	8,9	1,16 (0,38-3,54)	> 1,00
20. Fibrinosis greater than 5.0 g/l (for 2nd point of observation)	14	13,0	7	12,5	1,05 (0,39-2,78)	> 1,00
21. D-dimer levels over 500 ng/mL (2nd point of observation)	19	17,7	10	17,8	0,99 (0,42-2,31)	> 1,00
22. Herpes type 1 and 2	35	32,7	21	37,5	0,81 (0,41-1,59)	> 1,00
23. Hypothyroidism	6	5,6	4	7,1	0,77 (0,20-2,85)	0,737
24. Leukocytosis over 11,0×10^9/l (1st point of observation)	23	21,5	15	26,8	0,74 (0,35-1,58)	> 1,00
25. Blood group - is not "0"	85	79,4	47	83,9	0,74 (0,31-1,73)	0,535
26. Polymorphism of MTHFR (C/T, T/T)	30	28,0	23	41,0	0,55 (0,28-1,10)	0,113
27. Mutation of FV Leiden (G/A)	1	0,9	1	1,7	0,51 (0,03-8,45)	> 1,00

Table 13. Factors contributing to the failure of pregnancy in IVF cycles in the 1 st. observation group (n = 163)

Criterion	Failure of IVF (n=61)		Success of IVF (n=63)		Odds ratio (0,95% CI)	P-value
	Abs	%	Abs	%		
1. Hyperstimulation (early stage)	12	19,6	0	0	32,0 (1,85-555)	< 0,0001
2. Oligozoospermia (moderate and severe)	26	42,6	4	6,3	10,9 (3,53-34,0)	0,0002
3. Insufficient number of embryos transferred in IVF cycles (1-2)	23	37,7	8	12,7	4,16 (1,68-10,28)	0,003
4. Homocysteine in blood of more than 15 nM/l (on the 1st point of observation)	14	22,9	5	7,9	3,45 (1,16-10,2)	0,043
5. Difficult embryo transfer	18	29,5	7	11,1	3,34 (1,28-8,74)	0,013
6. Mutation FII (G/A, A/A)	1	1,6	0	0	3,14 (0,12-78,8)	0,491
7. Defective embryo	17	27,8	8	12,7	2,65 (1,04-6,72)	0,044
8. Peak thrombin more than 360 mM/l (for 2nd point of observation)	43	70,4	32	50,8	2,31 (1,10-4,84)	0,028
9. ETP more than 1900 nM/min (2nd point of observation)	41	67,2	31	49,2	2,11 (1,02-4,38)	0,047
10. Unsuccessful IVF attempt in anamnesis	11	18,0	6	9,5	2,09 (0,72-6,06)	0,198
11. D-dimer levels over 500 ng/mL (2-nd point of observation)	13	21,3	8	12,7	1,86 (0,71-4,87)	0,476
12. Age (36-40 years)	8	13,1	5	7,9	1,75 (0,53-5,68)	0,392
13. Polymorphism of PAI-I (5 G/4 G, 4 G/4 G)	26	42,6	20	31,7	1,59 (0,76-3,32)	0,265
14. Cytomegalovirus infection	3	4,9	2	3,1	1,57 (0,25-9,78)	1,677
15. EAAF index less than 11% (1st point of observation)	33	54,0	27	42,8	1,57 (0,77-3,19)	0,280
16. The combination of polymorphisms MTHFR (C/T, T/T) and PAI-I (5 G/4 G, 4 G/4 G)	17	27,8	13	20,6	1,48 (0,64-3,40)	0,706
17. Fibrinosis greater than 5.0 g/l (for the 2nd point of observation)	8	13,1	6	9,8	1,43 (0,46-4,40)	0,580

Criterion	Failure of IVF (n=61)		Success of IVF (n=63)		Odds ratio (0,95% CI)	P-value
	Abs	%	Abs	%		
18. High-dose protocol	6	9,8	5	7,9	1,26 (0,36-4,38)	0,760
19. Blood group - is not "0"	48	78,6	47	74,6	1,24 (0,54-2,89)	0,673
20. Low ovarian reserve	11	18,0	10	15,8	1,16 (0,45-2,98)	0,813
21. Clot lysis time of over 12 minutes (1st point of observation)	35	57,4	34	53,9	1,14 (0,56-2,33)	0,720
22. Leukocytosis over 11,0×10⁹/l (1st point of observation)	13	21,3	12	19,0	1,15 (0,47-2,77)	0,824
23. Hypoplasia of the endometrium	4	6,5	4	6,3	1,03 (0,24-4,33)	> 1,00
24. Hypothyroidism	4	6,5	4	6,3	1,03 (0,24-4,33)	> 1,00
25. Herpes type 1 and 2	7	11,4	9	14,3	0,77 (0,27-2,23)	0,790
26. Polymorphism of MTHFR (C/T, T/T)	12	19,6	25	39,6	0,37 (0,16-0,83)	0,018

Table 14. Factors contributing to the failure of pregnancy in IVF cycles in the 2nd group (n = 124)

In our publication we studied a number of women with the known risk factors of IVF failures to be less significant regardless of the ongoing correction of hemostasis and hypo fibrinolysis. We also record such risk factors as manifestations of inflammatory reaction (leukocytosis, fibrinosis) of virus (herpes, cytomegalovirus), the pathology of the thyroid gland and a number of others.

We are particularly interested in the reasons for the failure of IVF which remained relevant after therapeutic correction aimed at hemostasis and fibrinolysis. The list is given in Table. 15.

As noted earlier (Table 14), in addition to gynecological risk factors, hyperhomocysteinemia, and manifestations of excessive thrombin generation became the causes of the failure of IVF. Consequently, despite treatment some female patients maintained the trend to intravascular coagulation. Earlier, Table 11 demonstrated that isolated course of IPC to treat hypo fibrinolysis and other effects led to increased thrombin generation whereas the combination of IPC with dalteparin did not lead to such a shift (Table 12). Considering that we used three variants of therapeutic intervention our attempt was to determine the frequency of each of them under different outcomes of IVF in women with a high ETP in thrombin generation test.

Criterion	Failure of IVF (n=56)		Success of IVF (n=42)		P-value
	Abs.	%	Abs.	%	
1. Hyperstimulation (early stage)	10	17,8	0	0	0,004
2. Oligozoospermia (moderate and severe)	22	39,3	4	9,5	< 0,001
3. Insufficient number of embryos transferred in IVF cycles (1-2)	18	32,1	5	11,1	0,029
4. Homocysteine in blood of more than 15 nM/l (on the 1st point of observation)	17	30,3	4	9,5	0,039
5. Difficult embryo transfer	19	33,9	6	14,2	0,035
6. Defective embryo	18	32,1	5	11,1	0,029
7. ETP more than 1900 nM/min (2nd point of observation)	39	69,6	17	40,5	0,006
8. Peak thrombin more than 360 mM/l (for 2nd point of observation)	42	75,0	19	45,2	0,003

Table 15. Causes for the failure of IVF under conducted therapeutic correction of hemostasis and fibrinolysis (n = 98)

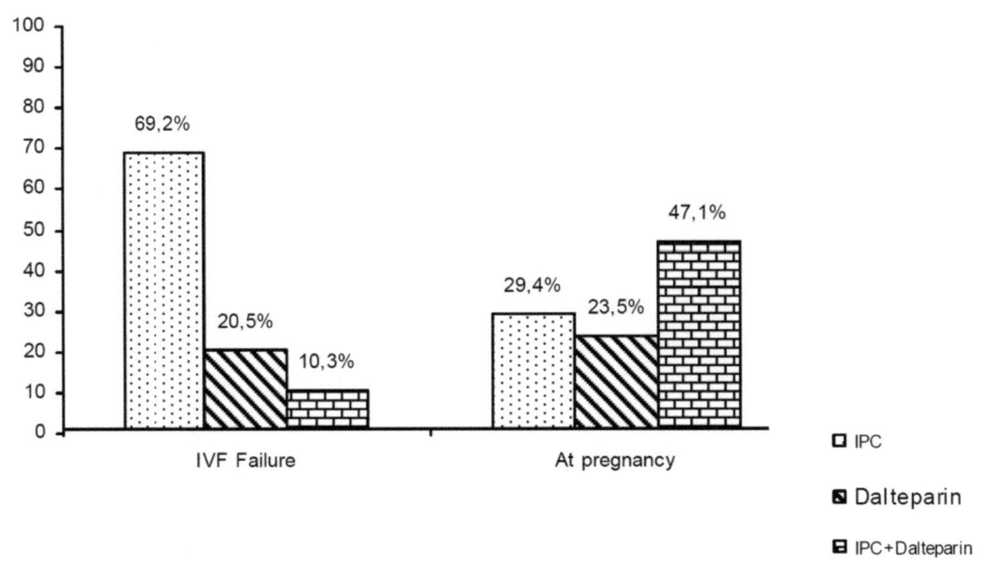

Figure 4. Analysis of the effectiveness of different therapies with excessive thrombin generation (ETP to 1900 nM/min in the 2nd point of observation)

The data in Figure 4 show that the high generation of thrombin and IVF failure is more common in the course of isolating IPC and less - in combination therapy.

6. Discussion

To sum up the results we note that excessive thrombin generation and a fibrinolytic inhibition fatal reaction (without correction) reduces the effectiveness of IVF and has a comparable value compared to the traditional risk factors of reproduction. Thus, our study proves a number of recent statements devoted to this problem (Martinez-Zamora et al., 2011; Meltzer et al., 2010; Nelson & Greer, 2008; Rova et al., 2012; Westerlund et al., 2012). However, we have made further progress due to suprathreshold values of laboratory parameters which allow to monitor the increased propensity to blood clotting and / or hypo fibrinolysis and therefore to identify patients with high risk of IVF failure in order to conduct therapeutic correction of disorders . In particular, by the calibrated test of thrombography administration of dalteparin was authorized by its indicators (ETP, Peack thrombin) to lead to the effective reduction of thrombin generation as well as the significant increase in positive outcomes of IVF (6.4 times).

We first proposed and tested method and mode of correction hypo fibrinolysis IPC for women in a cycle of IVF. It was shown that vases compression in these cases leads to the increased activity of t-PA and reduced PAI-1 activity, which is clearly manifested by the sharp increase in the calculated EAAF index , accelerated clotlysis time and the increase in the number of positive outcomes for assisted reproductive technology in 3 times. However, there were no obvious reasons to reduce the dynamic activity of PAI-1 during the course of IPC, even though it appeared to be a favorable result of the non-drug therapy. A negative consequence of the IPC was the phenomenon increasing the generation of thrombin which did not have the prior record. The calculations showed that the IPC in all cases should be combined with heparin prophylaxis to obtain the best clinical results. In this publication, combining vases compression with prophylactic doses of LMWH (low molecular weight heparin) really helped to increase the number of pregnancies in 6.5 times. In our opinion, this non-pharmacological approach to correcting hypo fibrinolysis demonstrates great potential for use in a number of clinical situations, including pregnancy period. In this chapter, we do not include the results of vases compression in women with low fibrinolytic activity after IVF in the first 12 weeks of pregnancy. However, the results are encouraging and will be published later.

The leading role of increased thrombin generation and hypo fibrinolysis in negative consequences of this reproductive technology has been proved in comparative evaluation of the significance of the risk factors of IVF failure. Its value appeared to be comparable with such risk factors as ovarian hyperstimulation syndrome, male factor, poor embryo or small quantities, or hard to bear embryos. In the meantime, the range of risk factors and their significance has changed dramatically after the treatment and correction of disorders of hemostasis and fibrinolysis. In particular, the list of relevant factors was reduced significantly to hypo fibrinolysis (rated by EAAF index) whereas indicators of excessive thrombin generation remained, though in less prominent positions. In addition, risk factors such as male factor, insufficient and difficult embryo transfer, as well as their low quality became more significant. The publication indicates the important role of hyperhomocysteinemia in the failure of IVF. As you know, it refers to the controllable risk factors which can and must be eliminated by recognized medical methods (by taking vitamins B6, B12, folic acid) at pre-gravid preparation.

In our research, we tested only 7 women with rare mutations F V Leiden (1691 G>A) and FII (20210 G>A), associated with thrombosis, pregnancy failure and reproductive technologies. Therefore, we were unable to prove their relevance to IVF outcomes. A common gene polymorphisms MTHFR (C 677> T) and gene PAI 1 (5G>4G) compared with the results of Coulam and Jeyendran (2009b) did not prove the significance.

7. Conclusion

The research marks the opportunities to progress and improve outcomes of IVF based on the identification and correction of the pathology of hemostasis and fibrinolysis. The research data may serve as the basis for the development of guidelines and standards which allow improving the efficiency of modern reproductive technologies. The marked problem requires interdisciplinary approach, joint efforts by obstetricians and hematologists and reward by better efficiency of IVF despite the increased cost of diagnosis and treatment of disorders of hemostasis and fibrinolysis.

Author details

Andrey Momot, Lyudmila Tsyvkina and Galina Serdyuk
Russian Academy of Medical Sciences, Hematological Research Center, Altai Department, Russia

Inna Lydina and Oksana Borisova
Clinical Regional Hospital, Barnaul, Russia

8. References

Alviggi C, Humaidan P, Howles CM, Tredway D. & Hillier S.G. (2009) Biological versus chronological ovarian age: implications for assisted reproductive technology. Reprod Biol Endocrinol. 2009;22:101-13.

American Society for Reproductive Immunology Antiphospholipid Antibody Committee: A rational basis for antiphospholipid antibody testing and selective immunotherapy in assisted reproduction: a rebuttal to the American Society for Reproductive Medicine Practice Committee Opinion. Fertil Steril. 2000;74:631-4.

American Society of Reproductive Medcine. Birmingham. Alabama. Antiphospholipid Antibodies Do Not Affect IVF Success. Fertil Steril. 2008;90:S172-3.

Andersson O, Blombäck M, Bremme K. & Wramsby H. (1997) Prediction of changes in levels of haemostatic variables during natural menstrual cycle and ovarian hyperstimulation. Thromb Haemost 1997;77:901-4.

Anteby Y, Greenfield C. & Natanson-Yaron S. (2004) Vascular endothelial growth factor, epidermal growth factor and fibroblast growth factor-4 and -10 stimulate trophoblast plasminogen activator system and metalloproteinase-9. Mol. Hum Reprod. 2004;10:229-35.

Aune B, Hoie KE, Oian P, Holst N. & Osterud B. (1991) Does ovarian stimulation for in-vitro fertilization induce a hypercoagulable state? Hum Reprod 1991;6:925-7.

Azem F, Many A, Yovel I, Amit A, Lessing JB. & Kupfermic MJ. (2004) Increased rates of thrombophilia in women with repeated IVF failure. Hum Reprod. 2004;19:368- 70.

Balasch J, Miró F, Burzaco I, Casamitjana R, Civico S, Ballescá JL, Puerto B. & Vanrell JA. (1995) The role of luteinizing hormone in human follicle development and oocyte fertility: evidence from in vitro fertilization in a woman withlong-standing hypogonadotrophic hypogonadism and using recombinant human follicle stimulating hormone. Hum Reprod. 1995;10:1678-83.

Баркаган З.С., Момот А.П. Диагностика и контролируемая терапия нарушений гемостаза. / М., Изд-во: "Ньюдиамед-АО", 2001. - 296 С.

Bates SM, Greer IA, Pabinger I, Sofaer S. & Hirsh J. (2008) Venous Thromboembolism, Thrombophilia, Antithrombotic Therapy, and Pregnancy American College of Chest Physicians Evidence-Based Clinical Practice Guidelines (8th Edition). Chest. 2008;133:844-86.

Beer AE, Kwak J. (2000) Reproductive medicine program Finch University of I lealth Science. Chicago Med School. 2000;96.

Bellver J, Soares SR, Alvarez C, Muñoz E, Ramirez A, Rubio C, Remohi J. & Pellicer A. (2008) The role of trombophilia and thyroid autoimmunity in unexplained infertility, implantation failure and recurrent spontaneous abortion. Hum Reprod. 2008;23(2):278-84.

Berkarda B, Akokan G. & Derman U. (1965) Self-coagulogram. Thromb Diath Haemorrh. Mar. 1965; 15(13):297-303.

Berker B, Kaya C, Aytac R. & Satiroglu H. (2009) Homocystein concentrations in follicular fluid are associated with poor oocyte and embryo qualities in polycystic ovary syndrome patients undergoing assisted reproduction. Hum Reprod. 2009;24(9):2293-302.

Bertina R.M. (1997) Factor V Leiden and other coagulation factor mutations affecting thrombotic risk (1997) Clin Chem. 1997;43(9):1678-83.

Bertina RM, Koeleman BP, Koster T, Rosendaal FR, Dirven RJ, de Ronde H, van Velden PA. & Reitsma PH. (1994) Mitation in blood coagulation factor V associated with resistance to activated protein C. Nature. 1994;369(6475):64-7.

Birkenfeld A, Mukaida T, Minichiello L, Jackson M, Kase NG. & Yemini M. (1994) Incidence of autoimmune antibodies in failed embryo transfer cycles. Am J Repro Immunol. 1994;31(2-3):65-8.

Biron C, Galtier-Dereure F, Rabesandratana H, Bernard I, Aguilar-Martinez P, Schved JF. & Hedon B. (1997) Hemostasis parameters during ovarian stimulation for in vitro fertilization: results of a prospective study. Fertil Steril. 1997;67(1):104-9.

Bischof P, Aplin JD, Bentin-Ley U, Brannstrom M, Casslen B, Castrillo JL, Classen-Linke I, Critchley HO, Devoto L, D'Hooghe T, Horcajadas JA, Groothuis P, Ivell R, Pongrantz I, Macklon NS, Sharkey A, Vicovac L, White JO, Winterhager E, von Wolff M, Simon C. & Stavreus-Evers A. (2006) Implantation of the human embryo: Research lines and models. From the implantation Research Network 'Fruitful'. Gynecol Obstet Invest. Jun. 2006;62(4):206-16.

Bjornsson TD, Schneider DE. & Berger H. (1989) Aspirin acetylates fibrinogen and enhances fibrinolysis. Fibrinolytic effect is independent of changes in plasminogen activator levels. J Pharmacol Exp Ther. 1989;250:154-61.

Bouma BN, Meijers JC. (2003) Thombin-activatable fibrinolysis inhibitor (TAFI, plasma procarboxypeptidase B, procarboxypeptidase R, procarboxypectidase U). Thromb Haemost. 2003;1: 1566-74.

Browse NL, Gary L, Jarrett PEM. & Morland M. (1977) Blood and vein-wall fibrinolytic activity in health and vascular disease. Br Med J. 1977;1:478-81.

Buchholz T, Lohse P, Rogenhofer N, Kosian E, Pihusch R. & Thaler CJ. (2003) Polymorphisms in the ACE and PAI-1 genes are associated with recurrent spontaneous miscarriages. Hum Reprod. 2003;18(11):2473-7.

Canonico M, Olie V, Carcailon L, Tubert-Bitter P. & Scarabin P-Y. on behalf of the Estrogen and Thromboembolism Risk (ESTHER) Study Group (2008) Synergism between non-O blood group and oral estrogen in the risk of venous thromboembolism among postmenopausal women: The ESTHER study. Thromb Haemost. 2008; 99(1):246-8.

Chan WS, Dixon ME. (2008) The "ART' of thromboembolism: A review of assisted reproductive technology and thromboembolic complications. Thromb Res. 2008:121:713-26.

Chouhan V, Comerota AJ, Sun I, Harada R, Gaughan JP. & Rao AK. (1999) Inhibition of tissue factor pathway inhibitor during intermittent pneumatic compression: a possible mechanism for antithrombotic effect. Arterioscler Thromb Vasc Biol. 1999; 19:2812-7.

Christen Y, Wutschert R, Weimer D, de Moerloose P, Kruithof EK. & Bounameaux H. (1997) Effects of intermittent pneumatic compression on venous haemodynamics and fibrinolytie activity. Blood Coagul Fibrinolysis. 1997;8:185-90.

Christiansen OB, Nielsen HS. & Kolte AM. (2006) Future directions of failed implantation and recurrent miscarriage research. Reprod Biomed Online. 2006;13:71-83.

Coulam C, Roussev R. (2009a) Antiphospholipid antibodies inhibit angiogenesis. Am J Reprod Immunol. 2009;81(2):149.

Coulam CB, Jeyendran D. (2009b) Trombophilic gene polymorphisms are risk factors for unexplained infertility. Fertil Steril 2009b;91(4):1516-7.

Coulam CB, Jeyendran RS, Fishel LA. & Roussev R. (2006a) Multiple thrombophilic gene mutations are risk factors for implantation failure. Reprod BioMed Online. 2006a;12:322-7.

Coulam CB, Jeyendran RS, Fishel LA. & Roussev RG. (2006b) Multiple thrombophilic gene mutations rather than specific gene mutations are risk factors for recurrent miscarriage. Am J Reprod Immunol. 2006b; 55:360-8.

Curnow JL, Morel-Kopp M-C, Roddie C, Aboud M. & Ward CM. (2006) Reduced fibrinolysis and increased fibrin generation can be detected in hypercoagulable patients using the overall hemostatic potential assay. Thromb Haemost. 2006;5:528-34.

Current Practices and Controversies in Assisted Reproduction. Report of a meeting on «Medical, Ethical and Social Aspects of Assisted Reproduction» held at WHO Headquarters in Geneva, Switzerland, 17-21 Sept 2001. WHO, Geneva, 2002:396 P.

Curvers J, Nap AW, Thomassen MC, Nienhuis SJ, Hamulyak K, Evers JL, Tans G. & Rosing J. (2001) Effect of in vitro fertilization treatment and subsequent pregnancy on the protein C pathway. Br J Haematol. 2001;a115:400-7.

Dahlbäck B, Carlsson M. & Svensson PJ. (1993) Familial thrombophilia due to a previously unrecognized mechanism characterized by poor anticoagulant response to activated protein C: prediction of cofactor to protein C. Proc Natl Acad Sci U.S.A. 1993;90(3):1004-8.

Damti OB, Sarid O, Sheiner E, Zilberstein. & Cwikel J. (2008) Stress and distress in infertility among women. Harefuah. 2008;147(3):256-60.

Dargaud Y, Hierso S, Rugeri L, Battie C, Gaucherand P, Négrier C. & Trzeciak MC. (2010) Endogenous thrombin potential, prothrombin fragment 1 + 2 and D-dimers during pregnancy. Thromb Haemost. 2010; 103(2):469 -71.

Dmowski WP, Rana N, Michalowska J, Friberg J, Papesirniak C. & El-Roeiy A. (1995) The effect of endometriosis, its stage and activity and of autoantibodies on in vitro fertilization/ Embryo Transfer Success Rates. Fertil Steril. 1995;63:555-62.

Ebish IM, Thomas CM, Wetzels AM, Willemsen WN, Sweep FC. & Steegers-Theunissen RP. (2008) Review of the role of the plasminogen activator system and vascular endothelial growth factor in subfertility. Fertil Steril. Dec. 2008;90(6):2340-50.

Egbase PE, Al Sharhan M, Diejomaoh M. & Grudzinskas JG. (1999) Antiphospholipid antibodies in infertile couples with two consecutive miscarriages after in-vitro fertilization and embryo transfer. Hum Reprod. 1999;14(6):1483-6.

Friedler S, Zimerman A, Schachter M, Raziel A, Strassburger D. & Ron El R. (2005) The midluteal decline in serum estradiol levels is drastic but not deleterious for implantation after in vitro fertilization and embryo transfer in patients with normal or high responses. Fertil Steril. 2005;83:54- 60.

Geerts W, Selby R. (2003) Prevention of venous thromboembolism in the ICU. Chest. 2003;124:357S-63S.

Gelbaya TA, Tsoumpou I, Nardo LG (2009). "The likelihood of live birth and multiple birth after single versus double embryo transfer at the cleavage stage: a systematic review and meta-analysis". Fertil. Steril. 2009;94(3): 936-45.

Girolami A, Vianello F. (2000) The significance or nonsignificance of the G to A 2010 prothrombin polymorphism. Clin Appl Thromb Hemost. 2000;6:239-40.

Gleicher N, Vidali A. & Karande V. (2002) The immunological «Wars of the Roses»: disagreemants amongst reproductive immunologists. Hum Reprod. 2002;17:539-42.

Gordon H, Elie A, David D. & Holger J. (2012) Antithrombotic Therapy and Prevention of Thrombosis, 9th ed: American College of Chest Physicians Evidence-Based Clinical Practice Guidelines. Chest. 2012; 141(2Suppl):7S-47S.

Grandone E, Colaizzo D, Lo Bue A, Checola MG, Cittadini E. & Margaglione M. (2001) Inherited thrombophilia and in-vitro fertilization implantation failure. Fertil Steril. 2001;176:201-2.

Gregory L. (1998) Ovarian markers of implantation potential in assisted reproduction. Hum Reprod.1998;13:117-32.

Harris E, Pierangeli S. (2008) Primary, secondary and catastrophic antiphospholipid syndrome: what's in a name. Semin Thromb Hemost. 2008;34:219-26.

Heit J.A. (2007) Thrombophilia: clinical and laboratory assessment and management. Consultative Hemostasis and Thrombosis. - 2nd ed. Philadelphia, PA: Saunders Elsevier, 2007;213-44.

Hemker HC, Giesen P, Al Dieri R, Regnault V, de Smedr E, Wagenvoord R, Lecompte T. & Béguin S. (2003) Calibrated automated thrombin generation measurement in clotting plasma. Pathophysiol Haemost Thromb. 2003;33:4-15.

Hemker HC, Giesen PLA, Ramjee M, Wagenvoord R. & Béguin. (2000) The thrombogramm: Monitoring thrombin generation in platelet-rich plasma. Thromb Haemost. 2000;83(4):589-91.

Hemker HC Al Dieri R, De Smalt F. & Beguin S. (2006) Thrombin generation, a function test of the haemostatic-thrombotic system. Thromb Haemost 2006;96(5):553-61;

Hillier S.G. (1994) Current concepts of the roles of follicle stimulating hormone and luteinizing hormone in folliculogenesis. Hum Reprod. 1994;9:188-91.

Holemans R. (1963) Increase in fibrinoiytic activity by venous occlusion. J Appl Physiol. Nov. 1963;18:1123-9.

Howles CM, Kim CH. & Elder K. (2006) Treatment strategies in assisted reproduction for women of advanced maternal age. Int Surg. 2006;91:S37-S54.

Hull M, Corrigan E, Piazzi A. & Loumaye E. (1994) Recombinant human luteinizing hormone: an effective new gonadotropin preparation. Lancet. 1994;344:334-5.

International Committee for Monitoring Assisted Reproductive Technology (ICMART), de Mouzon J, Lancaster P, Nygren KG, Sullivan E, Zegers-Hochschild F, Mansour R, Ishihara O. & Adamson D. (2009) World collaborative report on assisted reproductive technology, 2002. Hum Reprod. Sep;2009;24(9):2310-20.

Jacobs DG, Piotrowski JJ, Hoppensteadt DA, Salvator AE. & Fareed J. (1996) Hemodynamie and fibrinolytie consequences of intermittent pneumatic compression: preliminary results. J Trauma. 1996; 40:710-6.

Januszko T, Reutt H, Malofiejew M. & Buluk K. (1967) Plasminogen activator in the course and after physical exercise. Acta Physiol Pol. 1967;18:272-9.

Jerzak M, Putowski L. & Baranowski W. (2003) Homocystein level in ovarian follicular fluid or serum as predictor of successful fertilization. Ginekol Pol. 2003;74(9):949-52.

Kakkos SK., Nicolaides AN, Griffin M. & Geroulakos G. (2005) Comparison of two intermittent pneumatic compression systems. A hemodynamic study. International Angiology. 2005;24(4):330-5.

Keber D, Stegnar M, Keber I. & Acceito B. (1979) Influence of moderate and strenuous daily physical activity on fibrinolytic activity of blood: possibility of piasminogen activator stores depletion. Thromb Haemost. 1979;41:745-55.

Kim DK, Kim JW, Kim S, Gwon HC, Ryu JC, Huh JE, Choo JA, Choi Y, Rhee CH. & Lee WR. (1997) Polymorphism of angiotensin converting enzyme gene is associated with circulating levels of plasminogen activator inhibitor-1. Arterioscler Thromb Vasc Biol. 1997;17(11):3242-7.

Kim HC, Kemmann E, Shelden RM. & Saidi P. (1981) Response of blood coagulation parameters to elevated endogenous 17 beta-estradiol levels induced by human menopausal gonadotropins. Am J Obstet Gynecol. 1981;140:807-10.

Knight MTN, Dawson R. (1976) Effect of intermittent compression of the arms on deep venous thrombosis in the legs. Lancet. 1976; 2:1265-7.

Kowarzyk H, Buluk K. (1954) Trombina, proteasa trombinowa i plazmina. Acta physiol Pol. 1954;5(1):35-56.

Ku SY, Kim SD, Jee BC, Suh CS, Choi YM, Kim JG, Moon SY. & Kim SH. (2006) Clinical efficacy of body mass index as predictor of in vitro fertilization and embryo transfer outcomes. J Korean Med Sci. 2006;21:300-3.

Lazarus JH, Premawardhana LD. (2005) Screening for thyroid disease in pregnancy. J Clin Pathol. 2005;58:449-52.

Lintsen AME, Eijkemans MJC, Hunault CC, Bouwmans CAM, Hakkaart L, Habbema JDF. & Braat DDM Predicting ongoing pregnancy chances after IVF and ICSI: a national prospective study. Hum Reprod. 2007;22(9):2455-62.

Lintsen AM, Pasker-de Jong PC, de Boer EJ, Burger CW, Jansen CA, Braat DD. & van Leeuwen FE. (2005) Effects of subfertility cause, smoking and body weight on the success rate of IVF. Hum Reprod. 2005;20(7):1867-75.

Lisman T, Leebek FWG, Meijer K, Van Der Meer J, Nieuwenhuis K. & De Groot P. (2002) Recombinant factor VIIa improves clot formation but not fibrinolytic potential in patients with cirrhosis and during liver transplantation. Hepatology. 2002;35:616-21.

Lisman T, deGroot PG, Meijers JCM. & Rosendaal FR. (2005) Reduced plasma fibrinolytic potential is a risk for venous thrombosis. Blood. 2005;105:1102-5.

Macdonald RL, Amidei C, Baron J, Weir B, Brown F, Erickson RK, Hekmatpanah J. & Frim D. (2003) Randomized, pilot study of intermittent pneumatic compression devices plus dalteparin versus intermittent pneumatic compression devices plus heparin for prevention of venous thromboembolism in patients undergoing craniotomy. Surg Neurol. 2003;59(5):363-72.

Macey MG, Bevan S, Alam S, Verghese L, Agrawal S, Beski S, Thuraisingham R. & MacCallum PK. (2010) Platelet activation and endogenous thrombin potential in preeclampsia. Thromb Res. 2010;125(3):e76-e81.

Maheshwari A, Hamilton M. & Bhattchary S. (2008) Effect of female age on the diagnostic categories of infertility. Hum Reprod. 2008;23(3):538-42.

Many A, Schrieber L, Rosner S, Lessing JB, Eldor A. & Kupferminc MJ. (2001) Pathologic features of the placenta in women with severe pregnancy complications and thrombophilia. Obstet Gynecol. 2001;98(6):1041-4.

Margalioth E, Ben-Chetrit A, Gal M. & Eldar-Geva T. (2006) Investigation and treatment of repeated implantation failure following IVF-ET. Hum Reprod. 2006;21(12):3036-43.

Martinez-Zamora MA, Creus M, Tassies D, Reverter JC, Civico S, Carmona F. & Balasch J. (2011) Reduced plasma fibrinolytic potential in patients with recurrent implantation failure after IVF and embryo transfer. Hum Reprod. 2011;26 (3):510-6.

Martınez-Zamora MA, Creus M, Tassies D, Bové A, Reverter JC, Carmona F. & Balasch J. (2010) Thrombin activatable fibrinolysis inhibitor and clot lysis time in women with recurrent miscarriage associated with the antiphospholipid syndrome. Fertil Steril. 2010;94:2437-40.

Matsubayashi H, Sugi, T, Arai T, Shida M, Kondo A, Suzuki T, Izumi, S. & McIntyre JA. (2006) IgG-antiphospholipid antibodies in follicular fluid of IVF-ET patients are related to low fertilization rate of their oocytes. Am J Reprod Immunol May 2006;55(5):341-8.

Mc Clamrock H.D. (2008) The great weight debate: do elevations in body mass index (BMI) exert a negative extraovarian effect on in vitro fertilization outcome? Fertil Steril. 2008;89:1609-10.

Megan L, Meike L, Uhter H, Edward G, John J, Kevin J. & Angeline N. (2008) Body Mass Index: Impact on IVF Success Appears. Hum Reprod 2008;23:1835-9.

Meltzer ME, Doggen CJ, de Groot PG, Rosendaal FR. & Lisman T. (2009) Reduced plasma fibrinolytic capacity as a potential risk factor for a first myocardial infarction in young men. Br J Haematol. 2009;145:121-7.

Meltzer ME, Lisman T, De Groot PG, Meijers JCM, Le Cessie S, Doggen CJM. & Rosendaal FR. (2010) Venous thrombosis risk associated with plasma hypofibrinolysis is explained by elevated plasma levels of TAFI and PAI-1. Blood. 2010;116:113-21.

Navot D, Rosenwaks L. & Margalioth E. (1987) Prognostik assessment of female fecundity. Lancet. 1987;2:645-7.

Nelen W, Bulten J. & Steegers E. (2000) Maternal homocysteine and chorionic vascularization in recurrent early pregnancy loss. Hum Reprod. 2000;15:954-60.

Nelen WL, Blom HJ, Thomas CM, Steegers EA, Boers GH. & Eskes TK. (1998) Methylenetetrahydrofolate reductase polymorphism affects the change in homocysteine and folate concentrations resulting from low dose folic acid supplementation in women with unexplained recurrent miscarriages. J Nutrition. 1998;128:1336-41.

Nelson SM. (2009) Prophylaxis of VTE in women - during assisted reproductive techniques. Thromb Res. 2009;123:8-15.

Nelson SM, Greer IA (2008) The potential role of heparin in assisted conception. Hum Reprod. Update. Nov.-Dec. 2008;14:623-45.

Nyboe Andersen A, Goossens V, Bhattacharya S, Ferraretti AP, Kupka MS, de Mouzon J, Nygren KG. & The European IVF-monitoring (EIM) Consortium, for the European Society of Human Reproduction and Embryology (ESHRE). Assisted reproductive technology and intrauterine inseminations in Europe, 2005: results generated from European registers by ESHRE: ESHRE. The European IVF Monitoring Programme (EIM), for the European Society of Human Reproduction and Embryology (ESHRE). Hum Reprod 2009;24(6):1267-87.

Ohira T, Cushman M, Tsai MY, Zhang Y, Heckbert SR, Zakai NA, Rosamond WD. & Folsom AR. (2007) ABO blood group, other risk factors and incidence of venous thromboembolism: the Longitudinal Investigation of Thromboembolism Etiology (LITE). Thromb Haemost. 2007;5:1455-61.

Pandolfi M, Robertson B, Isacson S. & Niisson IM. (1968) Fibrinolytic activity of human veins in arms and legs. Thromb Diath Haemorrh. 1968;20:247-55.

Papanikolaou G, Evangelos G. 1, Kolibianakis E, Efstratios M, Tournaye H, Venetis CA, Fatemi H, Tarlatzis B. & Devroey P. (2008) Live birth rates after transfer of equal number of blastocysts or cleavage-stage embryos in IVF. A systematic review and meta-analysis. Hum Reprod. 2008;23(1):91-9.

Pioneers in in vivo Fertilisation. Ed. A.Th. Alberda, R.A. Gan, H.M. (1995) Vemer. London-New York:The Parthenon Publishing Group 1995;114.

Poort SR, Rosendaal FR, Reitsma PH. & Bertina RM. (1996) A common genetic variation in the 3- prime-untranslated region of the prothrombin gene is associated with elevated plasma prothrombin levels and an increase in venous thrombosis. Blood. 1996;88:3698-703.

Qublan H, Eid S. (2006) Acquired and inherited thrombophilia: implication in recurrent IVF and embryo transfer failure. Hum Reprod. 2006;21(10):2694-8.

Quenby S, Nik H, Innes B, Lash G, Turner M, Drury J. & Bulmer J. (2009) Uterine natural killer cells and angiogenesis in recurrent reproductive failure. Hum Reprod. 2009;24:45-54.

Regnault V, Beguin S. & Lecompte T. (2003) Calibrated automated thrombin generation in frozen-thawed platelrich plasma to detect hypercoagulability. Pathophysiol Haemost Thromb. 2003;33:23-9.

Rice VC, Richard-Davis G, Saleh AA, Ginsburg KA, Mammen EF, Moghissi K. & Leach R. (1993) Fibrinolytic parameters in women undergoing ovulation induction. Am J Obstet Gynecol. 1993; 169 (6):1549-53.

Ridker PM, Miletich JP, Buring JE, Ariyo AA, Price DT, Manson JE. & Hill JA. (1998) Factor V Leiden mutation as a risk factor for recurrent pregnancy loss. Annals of Internal Medicine. 1998;128:1000-3.

Rova K., Passmark H. & Lindqvist P.G. (2012) Venous thromboembolism in relation to in vitro fertilization: an approach to determining the incidence and increase in risk in successful cycles. Fertil Steril. (2012);97(1):95-100.

Saleh RA, Agarwal A, Sharma RK, Nelson DR. & Thomas Jr AJ. (2002) Effect of cigarette smoking on levels of seminal oxidative stress in infertile men: a prospective study. Fertil Steril. 2002; 78:491-9.

Salzman EW, McManama GP, Shapiro AH, Robertson LK, Donovan AS, Blume HW, Sweeney J, Kamm RD, Johnson MC & Black PM. (1987) Effect of optimization of hemodynamics on fibrinolytie activity and antithrombotic efficacy of external pneumatic calf compression. Ann Surg. 1987;206:636-41.

Sarto A, Rocha M, Martinez M. & Pasqualini R. (2000) Hypofibrinolysis and other hemostatic defects in women with antecedents of early reproductive failure. Medicina. 2000;60:441-7.

Scheffer GJ, Broekmans FJ, Looman CW, Blankenstein M, Fauser BC, teJong FH. & teVelde ER. (2003) The number of antral follicles in normal women with proven fertility is the best reflection of reproductive age. Hum Reprod. 2003;18:700-6.

Seghatchian MJ, Samama MM. & Hecker SP. (1996) Hypercoagulable states. Fundamental aspects, acquired disorders, and congenital thrombophilia. C.R.C. Press. Boca Raton e.a. 1996;462 P.

Sher G, Fisch JD, Maassarani G, Matzner W, Ching W. & Chong P. (2000) Antibodies to phosphatidylethanolamine and phosphatidylserine are associated with increased natural killer cell activity in non-male factor infertility patients. Hum Reprod. 2000;15(9):1932-6.

Stern C, Chamley L. (2006) Antiphospholipid antibodies and coagulation defects in women with implantation failure after IVF and miscarriage. Reprod Biomed Online. 2006;13:29-37.

Tan BK, Vandekerckhove P. & Kennedy R. (2005) Investigation and current management of recurrent IVF treatment failure in the UK. BJOG. 2005;112:773.

Tarnay TJ, Rohr PR, Davidson AG, Stevenson MM, Byars EF. & Hopkins GR. (1980) Pneumatic calf compression, fibrinolysis, and the prevention of deep venous thrombosis. Surgery. 1980;88:489-96.

Tchaikovski SN, van Vliet HA, Thomassen MC, Bertina RM, Rosendaal FR. Sandset PM, Frans M Helmerhorst FM, Tans G. & Rosing J. (2007) Effect of oral contraceptives on thrombin generation measured via calibrated automated thrombography. Thromb Haemost. 2007;98(6):1350-6.

Triplett D.A. (1989) Antiphospholipid antibodies and recurrent pregnancy loss. Am Reprod Immun. 1989;20:52-7.

Turpie AG, Gallus A, Beattie WS. & Hirsh J. (1977) Prevention of venous thrombosis in patients with intracranial disease by intermittent pneumatic ompression of the calf. Neurology. 1977;27:435-8.

Urman B, Ata B, Yakin K, Alatas C, Aksoy S, Mercan R,. & Balaban B. (2009) Luteal phase empirical low molecular weight heparin administration in patients with failed ICSI embryo transfer cycles: a randomized open-labeled pilot trial. Hum Reprod. Jul 2009;24(7):1640-7.

Urman B, Yakin K. & Balaban B. (2005) Recurrent implantation failure in assisted reproduction: how to counsel manage. A. General considerations and treatment options that may benefit the couple. Reproductive BioMedicine Online. 2005;11:382-91.

Weitz J, Michelsen J, Gold K, Owen J. & Carpenter D. (1986) Effects of intermittent pneumatic calf compression on postoperative thrombin and plasmin activity. Thromb Haemost. 1986;56:198-201.

Westerlund E, Henriksson P, Wallén H, Hovatta O, Wallberg KR. & Antovic http://www.sciencedirect.com/science/article/pii/S0049384811006189 - af0005 A. (2012) Detection of a procoagulable state during controlled ovarian hyperstimulation for in vitro fertilization with global assays of haemostasis. Thromb Res. Apr. 2012;46(4):417-25.

Wichers IM, Tanck MW, Meijers JC, Lisman T, Reitsma PH, Rosendaal FR, Büller HR. & Middeldorp S. (2009) Assessment of coagulation and fibrinolysis in families with unexplained thrombophilia. Thromb Haemost. 2009;101:465-70.

Wielders S, Mukherjee M, Michiels J, Rijkers DT, Cambus JP, Knebel RW, Kakkar V, Hemker HC. & Béguin S. (1997) The routine determination of the endogenous thrombin potential, first results in different forms of hyper- and hypocoagulabillity. Thromb Haemost. 1997;77(4):629-36.

Younis JS, Brenner B, Ohel G, Tal J, Lanir N. & Ben-Ami M. (2000) Activated protein C resistance and factor V Leiden mutation can be associated with first-as well as second-trimester recurrent pregnancy loss. Am J Reprod Immunol. 2000;43(1):31-5.

Zorio E, Gilabert-Estellés J, España F, Ramón LA, Cosin R. & Estellés A. (2008) Fibrinolysis: the key to new pathogenetic mechanisms. Curr Med Chem. 2008;15:923-9.

Chapter 5

Intracytoplasmic Sperm Injection – Factors Affecting Fertilization

Murid Javed and Essam Michael

Additional information is available at the end of the chapter

http://dx.doi.org/10.5772/50036

1. Introduction

The ICSI has become method of choice to achieve fertilization. Fertilization is possible in cases in which the sperm motility and ability to penetrate the zona pellucida are impaired. Injection is possible with sperm obtained from ejaculation, microsurgical epididymal sperm aspiration (MESA), percutaneous epididymal sperm aspiration (PESA), or testicular sperm extraction (TESE). In addition, indications for ICSI include idiopathic infertility and repeated conventional *in vitro* fertilization (IVF) failures [1]. Fertilization rate after ICSI is at about 70 to 80% in all ages combined [2]. This suggests that, despite injecting sperm into mature oocytes, failed fertilization still occurs. Total failed fertilization (TFF) refers to failure of fertilization in all mature oocytes and "failed fertilization" refers to failure of fertilization in any mature oocyte. Based on a considerable emotional and financial involvement in a cycle of assisted reproduction, TFF is a distressful event for the infertile couple as well as the fertility professionals. TFF occurs in 5–10% of IVF [3] and 1-3% of ICSI cycles [4]. TFF after ICSI cycles is mostly due to low number of mature oocytes [4] or oocyte activation failure [5]. TFF is a rare event in cases with normal oocytes and sperm [6]. Some patients may face repeated TFF in spite of normal sperm parameters and good ovarian response [7]. In such cases, the primary reason for failed fertilization after ICSI is lack of oocyte activation, as more than 80% of these oocytes contain a sperm [4]. Considerable advances in artificial oocyte activation and recovery of sperm from epididymis or testis, suitable for ICSI, help avoid TFF. This chapter discusses the factors affecting success rate of ICSI, highlights causes of failure and suggests remedies for failed fertilization after clinical ICSI.

2. Procedural effects of ICSI technique

The risk of oocyte damage by the ICSI procedure is low in humans and is due to both the skill of the person performing the injection procedure and the quality of the gametes used during the procedure [8]. The embryologist performing ICSI procedure is a significant predictor of fertilization, and laboratory conditions (i.e. incubators, culture of oocytes individually versus grouped) do not affect the rates [9]. When fertilization failure in most or all of the injected oocytes occurs, with experienced practitioners using normal sperm, the diagnosis falls to oocyte dysfunction, oocyte activation failure, or inability of sperm to be decondensed and processed by the oocyte.

Although ICSI is now a routine, it remains a very demanding technique to master, due partly to its inherent technical difficulty and partly to the heterogeneity of the cases. It is generally agreed that the ICSI procedure is subject to a "learning curve" [9] and that one common technical failure is not depositing the sperm within the oocyte cytoplasm. In this situation, the oocyte membrane may not have been broken during attempts to aspirate the ooplasm into the ICSI needle. Thus, the sperm is deposited next to the membrane so that when the oolemma returns to its original position, the sperm is pushed out into the perivitelline space, or is trapped inside a sac formed by the membrane [10]. The sperm may also become adherent to the tip of the injection needle or remain within the injection needle and be inadvertently pulled out upon withdrawal of the needle from the cytoplasm. Aspiration of the ooplasm is always used to make sure that the oocyte membrane is broken during injection. However, if the ooplasm is aspirated too much, degeneration of the oocyte frequently results. The degeneration of oocytes after ICSI is often a result of a fault in the ICSI technique, e.g. an injection pipette that is too large, not positioned properly or not sharp enough. **Figure 1** shows different stages of egg maturation and damaged oocytes after ICSI and **Figure 2** shows normal and abnormal fertilization after ICSI.

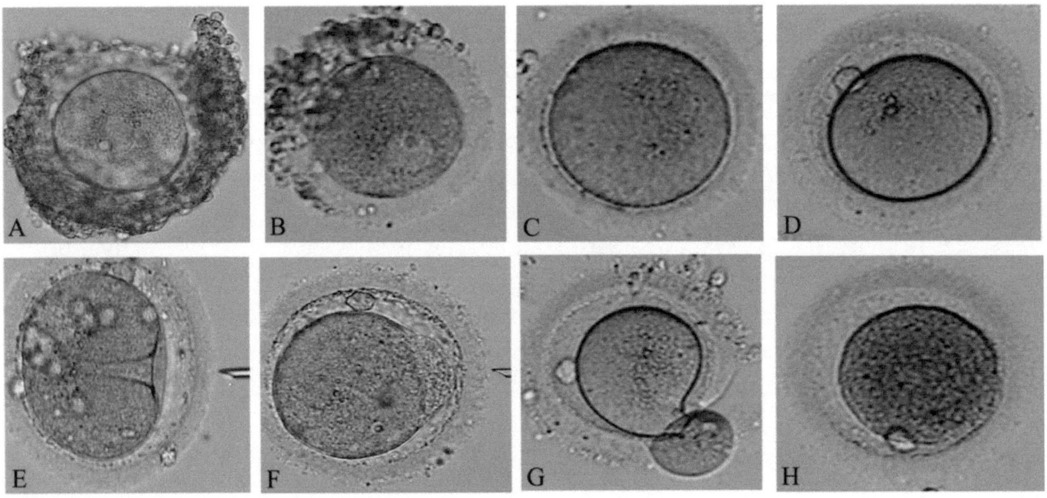

Figure 1. First row: A and B are GV, C is MI and D is MII oocyte. Second row: E shows typical funnel that appears after ICSI, F shows leakage of ooplasm after ICSI, G shows oocyte damage during denudation and H is an atretic oocyte after ICSI.

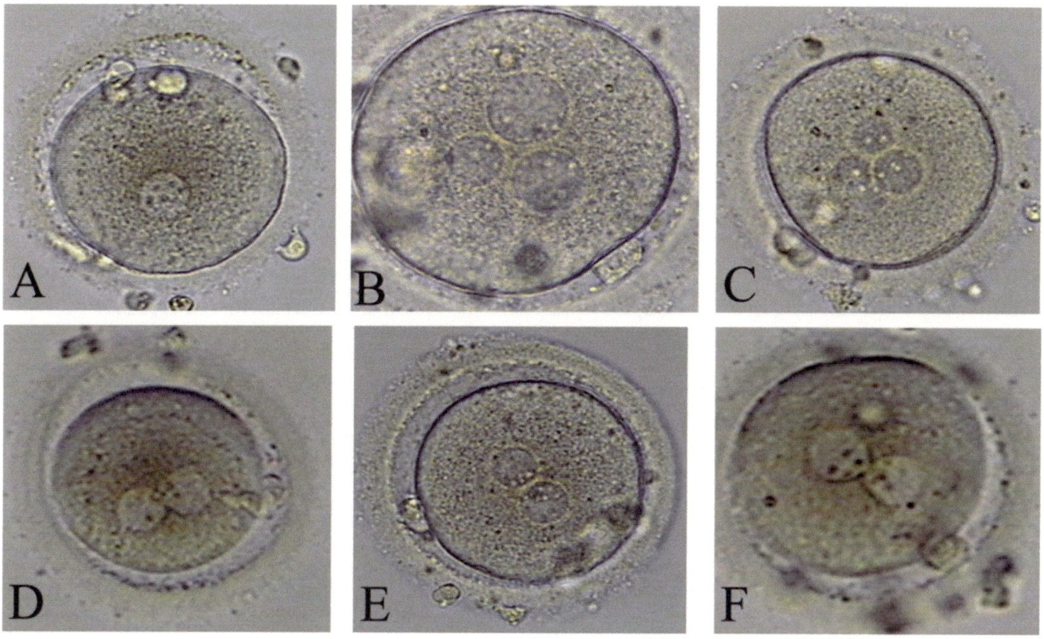

Figure 2. First row: A is an egg with1 pronucleus (PN), B with 3 and C with 4 PN. All these are abnormal fertilizations. Second row: Oocyte in D, E or F, each has 2 PN. This is a sign of normal fertilization.

Proper orientation of the polar body and needle position are also important, since improper positioning can damage or disrupt the metaphase plate during needle entry. In addition, disturbances in the nuclear spindle may dispose oocytes to aneuploidy or maturation arrest. Thus, perturbation of the cytoskeletal integrity of oocyte may critically influence the fate of the embryo. During ICSI, the location of the first polar body is commonly used as an indication of the spindle position, with the assumption that they are located in close proximity. To avoid damage to the spindle, oocytes are injected at the 3 o'clock position with the first polar body at the 6 or 12 o'clock position. However, with the aid of the computer assisted polarization microscopy, some reports suggest that the location of the first polar body does not necessarily correspond to the spindle position [11, 12]. The reasons for the displacement of the spindle are not fully understood [13]. Further detail on this aspect is given under use of Polscope.

Injection of a motile sperm without immobilization leads to poor fertilization rates [14]. In such cases, sperm with moving tails can be seen in the oocyte and sperm-oocyte interaction is obstructed by the normal sperm plasma membrane. Damage to the sperm membrane is necessary for successful oocyte activation following ICSI, as it induces gradual disruption of other parts of the sperm membrane allowing entry of sperm nucleus decondensing factor of the oocyte to induce initial swelling of the head. Because of this swelling, the sperm plasma membrane ruptures and sperm-associated oocyte activating factors are released into the ooplasm and induce oocyte activation. A modified ICSI technique is characterized by pushing the needle tip close to the membrane opposite the puncture site, aspirating the cytoplasm at this point and releasing the sperm in the centre of oocyte [5]. This modification improves fertilization in oocyte-dependent activation failure, but its routine application does not improve the overall results.

3. Use of PICSI

The cell surface hyaluronic acid (HA) binding glycoprotein is present in spermatozoa of different species including rat, mice, bull, and human [15]. The formation of hyaluronic-acid (HA)-binding sites on the sperm plasma membrane is one of the signs of sperm maturity. Various biochemical sperm markers indicate that human sperm bound to HA exhibit attributes similar to that of zona pellucida-bound sperm, including minimal DNA fragmentation, normal shape, and low frequency of chromosomal aneuploidies [16].

PICSI Sperm Selection Device (Biocoat, Inc. Horsham, PA, USA) offers advantage in selecting sperm for ICSI. The PICSI device, a dish similar to ICSI dish, contains 3 microdots of hyaluronan hydrogel which need to be hydrated by media before ICSI. The prepared sperm sample is placed at the edge of the microdrop of PICSI dish. Mature, biochemically competent sperm bind to the hyaluronan where they can be isolated by the embryologist and used for ICSI **(Figure 3)**. The research supports that hyaluronan-bound PICSI-selected sperm are, in the vast majority of cases, more mature, exhibit less DNA damage, and have fewer chromosomal aneuploidies [17]. Further studies are needed to prove that use of PICSI technique improves pregnancy rates and reduce the number of IVF miscarriages.

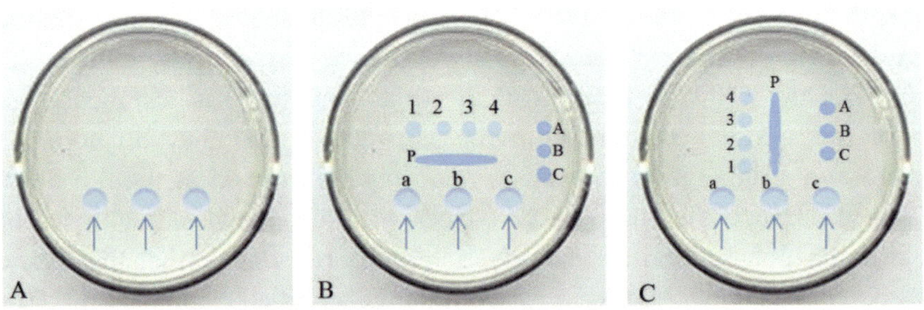

Figure 3. A is a graphical presentation of a PICSI dish. Each arrow is pointing to a dot containing hyaluronan. B and C are suggested arrangements for oocyte washing, PVP and ICSI drops (A, B and C are oocyte washing drops, P is PVP drop, a, b and c are hyaluronan dots and1, 2, 3, and 4 are ICSI drops).

4. Use of IMSI

Intracytoplasmic morphologically selected sperm injection (IMSI) is examination of unstained spermatozoa at 6000 or higher magnification to select sperm with best morphology. It is based on a method of high magnification motile sperm organelle morphology examination (MSOME) [18]. It requires an inverted light microscope equipped with high power Nomarski optics enhanced with digital imaging. Such examination helps to identify spermatozoa with a normal nucleus and nuclear content [19]. The exact indications of IMSI [20] and usefulness [21] are debatable. Finding normal-looking spermatozoa took a minimum of 60 min, and up to 210 min, depending on the quality of the semen sample. The technique required two embryologists working together on the analysis of the same sample at the same time in order to minimize the subjective nature of sperm evaluation [22]. The IMSI procedure improved embryo development and the laboratory and clinical outcomes of sperm microinjection in the same infertile couples with male infertility and poor embryo development over the previous ICSI attempts [23]. A successful childbirth after IMSI without assisted oocyte activation in a patient with globozoospermia has been reported [24]. Randomized large-scale trials are needed to confirm the beneficial effects of IMSI in couples with poor reproductive prognoses [25].

5. Use of polscope

The oocyte spindle can be imaged non-invasively based on the birefringence, an inherent optical property of highly ordered molecules, such as microtubules, as they are illuminated with polarized light. Polarized light microscopy has been applied to embryology for decades. A digital, orientation-independent polarized light microscope, the Polscope, has demonstrated the exquisite sensitivity needed to image the low levels of birefringence exhibited by mammalian spindles [26]. The Polscope, is used to protect the meiotic spindle from damage during ICSI. The oocytes having Polscope visualised spindle have higher fertilization rate. When the spindle is located at 0°-30° in relation to the first polar body, ICSI achieves highest fertilization rate [27]. The use of Polscope is still not widely practiced and further improvements are needed. Morphometric evaluation of the spindle through the Polscope is not consistent with confocal analysis. This suggests that the Polscope may still be a rather inefficient method for assessing the metaphase II spindle [28].

6. Timing of ICSI

Both nuclear and cytoplasmic maturation of oocytes have to be completed to ensure optimal conditions for fertilization. Oocytes are retrieved prior to ovulation for IVF or ICSI procedures. In the pre-ovulatory phase, meiotic division of the oocyte must progress to metaphase II which is considered nuclear maturation and is evident by extrusion of first polar body. The oocyte also must develop the capacity to attain fertilization and initiate embryo development which is considered cytoplasmic maturation [29, 30]. Cytoplasmic maturity is thought to be asynchronous with nuclear maturity in stimulated cycles [31, 32] and the fertilizing ability of an oocyte with a mature nucleus is not necessarily at its maximum potential. Thus, preincubation of oocytes prior to IVF or ICSI may induce cytoplasmic maturation that could eventually increase fertilization and also pregnancy rates. The human oocytes progressively develop the ability for full activation and normal development during the MII arrest stage [33].

The ICSI technique is generally similar among different centres but the time intervals from retrieval to denudation and from denudation to ICSI varies. Very few studies have addressed this aspect, with discrepancies in the conclusions [34, 35]. The preincubation period between oocyte retrieval and injection improves the percentage of mature oocytes [36, 37], the fertilization rate [35, 37], and the embryo quality [35]. The appropriate incubation time for mature oocytes before ICSI is 5–6 h. This time improves embryo quality and pregnancy rate in ICSI cycles. The maximum clinical pregnancy rate is observed when ICSI is performed 5 h after oocyte retrieval. The clinical pregnancy rate dropped significantly when ICSI was performed 6 hrs after oocyte retrieval (Falcone et al., 2008). A longer oocyte pre-incubation (9– 11 hours) prior to ICSI is thought to have detrimental effects on embryo quality [38], probably due to oocyte ageing.

7. Sperm related factors

7.1. Sperm structural defects

Normal sperm ultrastructure correlates with positive IVF results [39]. Single structural defects involving the totality of ejaculated sperm are among rare cases of untreatable human male infertility. This form of infertility is of genetic origin and is generally transmitted as an autosomal recessive trait. Numerous defective genes are potentially involved in human isolated teratozoospermia but such defects have not been defined at the molecular level in most cases [40]. An in-depth evaluation of sperm morphology by transmission electron microscopy (TEM) can improve the diagnosis of male infertility and can give substantial information about the fertilizing competence of sperm [41, 42]. The TEM evaluation of sperm can also identify potentially inheritable genetic disorders (for example primary ciliary dyskinesia, Kartagener's syndrome), providing valuable information for couples contemplating ICSI [43].

Abnormal spermatozoa with head vacuoles account for the patient infertility. Sperm head vacuoles are easily detectable in human spermatozoa under the electron microscope. A sperm head vacuole is considered abnormal when it exceeds 20% of the head's cross-sectional area. In rare cases, primary spermatozoa deformity is 100% vacuolated head [44]. There is a strong correlation between high relative vacuole area to sperm head and poor sperm morphology [45]. No correlation is observed between DNA defect and sperm-head morphology [46]. However, macrocephalic and large-headed spermatozoa are commonly associated with a low chance of pregnancy, mainly in relation to meiotic abnormalities during spermatogenesis. Enlarged-head spermatozoa are linked to sperm chromatin condensation dysfunction with no major meiotic dysfunction [47].

Acrosome agenesis is most often associated with a spherical shape of the head and is defined as "round head defect" or "globozoospermia". The underlying causes of the syndrome remain to be elucidated [48]. The genetic contribution has been postulated as well [49]. An additional case report [50] supports it. Studies show that the pathogenic genes associated with globozoospermia include SPATA16, PICK1, GOPC, Hrb, Csnk2a2 and bs

[51]. Globozoospermia results from perturbed expression of nuclear proteins or from an altered golgi-nuclear recognition during spermiogenesis. The sperm show both gross and ultrastructural abnormalities, including the complete lack of an acrosome, abnormal nuclear membrane and mid-piece defects. Depending on the severity of the defect, the fertilization rate after ICSI with round headed sperm ranges from 0% to 37% [52, 53]. Successful pregnancies have been reported after ICSI in patients with globozoospermia with or without oocyte activation [54, 53, 55]. The most likely cause for failed fertilization after ICSI using round-head sperm is inability of sperm to activate the oocyte. In some forms of globozoospermia, arrest of nuclear decondensation and/or premature chromosome condensation also causes fertilization failure [55].

7.2. Sperm DNA damage

DNA damage in the male germ line is associated with poor fertilization rates following IVF, defective pre-implantation embryonic development and high rates of miscarriage and morbidity in the offspring, including childhood cancer [56, 57]. Activation of embryonic genome expression occurs at the four to eight-cell stage in human embryos [58], suggesting that the paternal genome may not be effective until that stage. Therefore, a lack of correlation between elevated DNA strand breaks in sperm and fertilization rates may occur before the four to eight-cell stage [59, 60]. Many published articles indicate that DNA strand breaks are clearly detectable in ejaculated sperm and their presence is heightened in the ejaculates of men with poor semen parameters [61, 62]. Nuclear DNA damage in mature sperm includes single strand nicks and double strand breaks that can arise because of errors in chromatin rearrangement during spermiogenesis, abortive apoptosis and oxidative stress [63, 64]. In the same individuals, testicular samples show a significantly lower DNA damage compared to ejaculated spermatozoa (14.9%±5.0 vs. 40.6%±14.8, $P<0.05$), but significantly higher aneuploidy rates for the five analyzed chromosomes (12.41%±3.7 vs. 5.77%±1.2, $P<0.05$). While testicular spermatozoa appear favourable for ICSI in terms of lower DNA damage, this potential advantage could be offset by the higher aneuploidy rates in testicular spermatozoa [65].

Two tests are most commonly reported as indicators of sperm nuclear integrity; terminal deoxynucleotidyl transferase-mediated dUTP nick end labeling (TUNEL) and sperm chromatin structure assay (SCSA). The TUNEL technique labels single or double-stranded DNA breaks, but does not quantify DNA strand breaks in a given cell. The SCSA, a quantitative and flowcytometric test, measures the susceptibility of sperm nuclear DNA to acid-induced DNA denaturation *in situ*, followed by staining with acridine orange [66]. The SCSA accurately estimates the percentage of sperm chromatin damage expressed as DNA fragmentation index (DFI) with a cut-off point of 30% to differentiate between fertile and infertile samples [67]. A statistically significant difference is seen between the outcomes of ICSI versus IVF when DFI is >30% [68]. The biological explanation behind the superior results of ICSI in cases of high DFI needs to be elucidated. One possibility may be that women undergoing ICSI, on average, produce healthier oocytes with a better DNA repair capacity than women undergoing IVF, as in the ICSI group infertility is mainly caused by male factor.

Other tests of sperm nuclear DNA integrity include *in situ* nick translation and the comet assay. The toluidine blue and sperm chromatin dispersion test are potential new assays [69]. At present, there are two major strategies that may be considered for the treatment of men exhibiting high levels of DNA damage in their sperm: (i) selective isolation of relatively undamaged sperm and (ii) antioxidant treatment [70]. The lack of consensus in defining a clinically relevant standard DNA fragmentation test with a meaningful cut-off level brings challenges in implementing the routine use of sperm DNA integrity assessment in daily practice [71].

8. Injection with immature sperm

Round spermatid nucleus injection (ROSNI) or round spermatid injection (ROSI) is a method in which precursors of mature sperm obtained from ejaculated specimens or testicular sperm extraction (TESE) are injected directly into oocytes. ROSNI is proposed as a treatment for men in whom other more mature sperm forms (elongating spermatids or sperm) cannot be identified for ICSI [72]. It is not widely performed, not as successful as ICSI and is still an experimental procedure. It should be applied only in the setting of a clinical trial approved and overseen by a properly constituted institutional review board. Accurate identification of round spermatid is a technical challenge of ROSNI. It is difficult to distinguish haploid round spermatids from diploid spermatogenic precursors and somatic cells using the standard optics present in most clinical IVF laboratories. Mouse round spermatids have increased levels of DNA fragmentation [73] that may interfere with fertilization [63]. Increased DNA damage may occur because of deficient sperm nuclear protamine to histone replacement and decreased nuclear condensation in these immature sperm allowing increased susceptibility to reactive oxygen species and other damaging agents in culture. Another major concern is genetic risk. Any genetic abnormality sufficiently severe to result in meiotic arrest during spermatogenesis may also have adverse effects on other normal cellular processes or other systemic manifestations. Occurrence of significant congenital anomalies in ROSNI-conceived pregnancies raises serious concerns [74]. ROSNI should not be performed when more mature sperm forms (elongating spermatids or sperm) can be identified and used for ICSI. Patients who may be candidates for ROSNI should receive careful and thorough pre-treatment counselling to ensure they are clearly informed of the limitations and potential risks of the procedure [75].

9. Premature chromosomal condensation

When a cell, with chromosomes in MII, fuses with an inter-phase cell, the nuclear membrane of the cell in the inter-phase dissolves and its chromatin condenses. This phenomenon is called premature chromosomal condensation (PCC) [76]. Following penetration of sperm into an oocyte; oocyte activation is triggered, resulting in completion of meiosis and formation of both male and female pronuclei. Under some circumstances although the sperm is within the oocyte, fertilization fails to occur, the oocyte remains in the MII stage and the sperm head transforms into PCC, separate from the oocyte chromosomes [77, 78]. Chromatin analysis of human oocytes has revealed that sperm PCC is one of the prevalent causes of fertilization failure in both IVF and ICSI [77].

It is not yet fully understood how the sperm activates the oocytes. The failure of fertilization after ICSI may result from either the lack or deficiency of activating factors in sperm or from the lack of ooplasmic factors triggering sperm chromatin decondensation [79, 80]. Several pieces of evidence point to PLCζ being the physiological agent of oocyte activation and is detectable in different localities within the sperm head: the equatorial segment and acrosomal/post-acrosomal region [81].

During normal spermiogenesis, 85% of histones are replaced with protamines [82], which results in sperm chromatin condensation. A sperm with a condensed nucleus is in the G1 stage when entering an MII oocyte and is protected from PCC because an active maturation-promoting factor (MPF) is not capable of reacting with protamine-associated DNA. Once sperm nuclear decondensation factors from the ooplasm enter the sperm, the sperm head swells and sperm associated oocyte activating factor is released. This results in MPF inactivation [83], the completion of meiosis 2 and the oocyte enters the G1 stage. During this time, protamines are slowly replaced by histones and cell cycle synchronization takes place. Under some circumstances, the oocyte fails to activate and remains arrested at MII. Because of the presence of an active MPF, sperm chromatin transforms into condensed chromatin. Sperm with excessive histones are prone to PCC.

Sperm PCC has been associated with the type of ovarian stimulation protocol. Some protocols, such as clomiphene citrate and human menopausal gonadotropin stimulation may tend to recruit immature oocytes with immature cytoplasm [84]. Immature cytoplasm is believed to make sperm susceptible to a high incidence of PCC after insemination because of the inability of these immature oocytes to undergo oocyte activation [85]. The incidence of sperm PCC reported in the literature ranges from 10.1 to 85 % [86, 87], with higher values noted in cases of round headed sperm injection as they fail to activate the oocyte. Furthermore, other studies suggest a correlation between fertilization outcome post-ICSI and percentage of sperm with protamine deficiency [88]. The effect of sperm protamine deficiency on fertilization rate emphasizes the need for accurate sperm selection during ICSI as protamine-deficient sperm, in the form of slightly amorphous head, may find the chance of being injected due to inappropriate sperm selection [88].

10. Sperm motility and progression

Defective sperm tail is the principal cause of sperm motility disorders. There are two main forms of tail disorders with different phenotypic characteristics and consequences for male fertility: non-specific tail anomalies and various genetic disorders including primary ciliary diskinesia and the dysplasia of the fibrous sheath [89]. In non-specific tail anomalies, ICSI has good prognosis and does not pose additional risks in view of the lack of recognized genetic components in this Disorder. Significant sperm abnormalities of proven or suspected genetic origin are rare conditions responsible for extreme asthenozoospermia or total sperm immotility. Affected patients complain of male infertility and chronic respiratory disease, alterations caused by abnormal function of sperm flagella and respiratory cilia. In patients with tail genetic disorders, ICSI results in normal rates of fertilization and implantation, and many births of healthy babies have been reported. The main concern that remains is the potential transmission to the offspring [89].

Whether sperm movement is slow or rapid generally has no influence on ICSI results. However, injection of immotile sperm usually results in impaired fertilization. In particular, where a non-viable immotile sperm is injected into an oocyte, normal fertilization and pregnancy rarely occurs [90, 91]. In case of immotile sperm, it is possible that the sperm may be dead. The most common practice to select viable non-motile sperm for ICSI involves the hypo-osmotic swelling (HOS) test. However, preliminary results in animal experiments (mouse and rabbit) indicate that viability of injected sperm is not an absolute pre-requisite for fertilization. Embryos derived after injecting mouse oocytes with freeze-dried and thawed sperm developed normally [92]. It appears that provided the DNA integrity of the sperm is maintained, embryos can be generated, at least in animal model, from severely damaged sperm that are no longer capable of normal physiological activity.

The identification of a viable spermatozoon amongst immotile spermatozoa for ICSI often is difficult. However, selection of birefringent spermatozoa under Polscope shows promising results in asthenozoospermic men and men undergoing testicular sperm aspiration or extraction before ICSI [93]. The other tests employed are hypo-osmotic swelling test, the stimulation of motility with pentoxyfilline and non-contact diode laser [94, 95, 96, 97, 98].

In patients with 100% immotile sperm, HOS test is a useful method to examine sperm viability. It measures the functional integrity of the sperm membrane [99]. Upon exposure of the sperm to hypo-osmotic conditions, the intact semi-permeable barrier formed by the sperm membrane allows an influx of water and results in swelling of the cytoplasmic space and curling of the sperm tail fibers. Only viable sperm react to the HOS solution since dead sperm are unable to maintain the osmotic gradient.

Sperm HOS test based on fructose and sodium citrate dihydrate is applied for identification of immotile sperm for ICSI [100]. A significantly greater fertilization and cleavage rate after injection of sperm selected using the HOS test is achieved in contrast to injection of randomly selected sperm. A modified HOS test based on NaCl solution further improves fertilization rate in patients with 100% immotile sperm [101]. In these procedures, approximately 200,000 sperm are exposed to the HOS solution for 1 hour at 37°C. A modified HOS test has been used for samples with a low sperm count such as testicular samples [102]. In this technique, individual morphologically normal sperm is aspirated by microinjection pipette and is exposed to HOS solution for a brief period to minimize the sperm membrane damage.

A mixture of 50% culture medium and 50% deionized grade water has the least delayed harmful effects on sperm vitality [103]. This mixture achieves similar implantation, pregnancy and ongoing pregnancy rates in the ejaculated and testicular non-motile sperm groups [104]. It is a simple and practical procedure and achieves acceptable and comparable pregnancy rates.

Obtaining viable spermatozoa from testicular biopsies using pentoxifylline is more effective in terms of fertilization and pregnancies than obtaining it through an HOS test [97]. The clinical use of pentoxifylline for activation of immotile ejaculatory sperm before ICSI in patients with Kartagener's syndrome improves the outcome of the treatment and reduces the need of invasive intervention such as TESE in these patients. The immotile sperm are treated for 30 min with pentoxifylline (1.76 mM) before ICSI. Some spermatozoa show minimal motion and can be used for ICSI. Fertilization rate after ICSI is about 75% [105].

11. Sperm origin

A new era in the field of assisted reproduction opened after the achievement of pregnancies and births after ICSI of human oocytes [106]. In special cases of long-standing male infertility, only a few functional sperm are available. By means of ICSI, most sub-fertile men and even men previously considered sterile (those with azoospermia, extreme oligozoospermia or cryptozoospermia) can now father a child.

Azoospermia, is the most severe form of male factor infertility. The condition is currently classified as 'obstructive' or 'non-obstructive'. Obstructive azoospermia is the result of obstruction in either the upper or lower male reproductive tract. Sperm production may be normal but the obstruction prevents the sperm from being ejaculated. Non-obstructive azoospermia is the result of testicular failure where sperm production is either severely impaired or nonexistent, although in many cases sperm may be found and surgically extracted directly from the testicles [107].

Conflicting results for fertilization and pregnancy rates are available in the literature after use of ejaculated or surgically retrieved sperm. After ICSI, ejaculated or surgically extracted sperm, when motile and morphologically normal, result in similar fertilization, implantation [108, 109] and clinical pregnancy rates ([109]. The incidence of early or late spontaneous abortion and ectopic pregnancy, or malformations is also similar [108]. However, after conventional IVF, even testicular or epididymal aspirates with very good sperm concentration and motility, generally achieve low fertilization and pregnancy rates [110].

The effect of cryopreservation of sperm on ICSI outcome has been thoroughly studied. Current studies suggest that the use of fresh or frozen-thawed sperm does not appear to affect ICSI outcomes [111]. Testicular tissue and epididymal sperm can be cryopreserved successfully without markedly reducing subsequent fertilization and implantation rates and repeated testicular biopsy can be avoided without the risk of any decrease in the outcome [112].

The origin of the sperm used in ICSI does not have a major influence on the early life outcomes for the offspring, but transgenerational and epigenetic effects remain unknown. From the limited information available, it appears that there is no increased risk of congenital malformations in children born from ICSI. There is, however, a small increase in both de novo and inherited chromosome abnormalities. In terms of growth and neurodevelopment, there are very few studies, and so far, no adverse outcomes have been found in young children whose fathers have a sperm defect [113].

12. Oocyte related factors

12.1. Oocyte activation

Oocyte activation is a complex series of events that results in the release of the cortical granules, activation of membrane bound ATPase, resumption of meiosis with the extrusion of the second polar body and finally the formation of male and female pronuclei. The ovulated or retrieved oocyte activates when the sperm enters, by either natural penetration or ICSI. In cases of oocyte activation failure, artificial means of oocyte activation are helpful.

The oocytes remain arrested at MII if maturation has been completed. When one sperm contacts the oolemma and penetrates into the ooplasm, intracellular calcium oscillation occurs [114]. This increase in the concentration of calcium underlies oocyte activation and initiation of development. In mammals, growing experimental evidence supports the notion that, following fusion of the gametes, a factor from sperm is responsible for inducing calcium oscillations and stimulating inositol 1,4,5-trisphosphate (IP3) production [115]. Initial evidence stemmed from injection of cytosolic sperm extracts into oocytes that reproduced the calcium responses associated with fertilization regardless of the species of origin [116, 117]. Subsequent biochemical characterization of the extracts revealed that the active component contained a protein moiety [116] that possessed phospholipase C (PLC) - like activity capable of inducing production of IP3 [118, 119] and that the PLC activity was highly sensitive to calcium [120]. A screen of expressed sequenced tags from testes identified a sperm-specific phospholipase C, PLCζ. The presence of PLCζ correlates with calcium activity in cytosolic sperm extracts [121]. Moreover, injection of oocytes with the recombinant protein [122] or with the encoding mRNA induces fertilization-like oscillations (Saunders, 2002), whereas depletion of PLCζ from the extracts with specific antisera abrogates PLCζ activity [123] and the calcium oscillatory activity of the extracts [121, 123]. The PLCζ is located in the equatorial region of human sperm. Men whose sperm are unable to initiate calcium oscillations consistently fail to fertilize following ICSI and lack PLCζ [124]. It has to be established that PLCζ is the sole calcium oscillation–inducing factor and how its absence has an impact on male fertility.

The process of natural fertilization encompasses the entry of the sperm, oocyte activation and the first mitotic division resulting in a 2 cell embryo. Two steps are important for successful fertilization following ICSI, namely immobilization of the sperm and rupture of the oolemma in order to facilitate the liberation of the cytosolic sperm factor responsible for the oscillator function [14].

Low fertilization rates after ICSI in patients with round-headed sperm, globozoospermia, is a result of reduced ability of round-headed sperm to activate the oocyte. In the literature, the success rates of ICSI in cases of globozoospermia are variable. Assisted oocyte activation combined with ICSI may overcome the infertility associated with globozoospermia. Normal healthy live birth without assisted oocyte activation has also been achieved [54]. Apart from low fertilization rates associated with the use of round-headed sperm, cleavage rates are also compromised and these sperm may lack normal centrosomes [52]. Assisted oocyte activation and ICSI restore fertilization, embryo cleavage and development for patients with globozoospermia [125].

Assisted oocyte activation after ICS is very efficient in patients with a suspected oocyte-related activation deficiency and previous total fertilization failure after conventional ICSI. However, when there was a prior history of low fertilization, one should be careful and test the efficiency of assisted oocyte activation on half of the sibling oocytes, because assisted oocyte activation is not always beneficial for patients with previous low fertilization and a suspected oocyte-related activation deficiency. For these patients, a split assisted oocyte activation-ICSI cycle using sibling oocytes can help to distinguish between a molecular oocyte-related activation deficiency and a previous technical or other biological failure [126].

Assisted oocyte activation aims to mimic the action of sperm penetration [127]. Some assisted activation treatments such as strontium chloride [128] and ionomycin [129], promote an increase in intracellular free calcium concentrations by the release of calcium from cytoplasmic stores. Others such as electrical stimulus promote influx of calcium from the extracellular medium and some treatments such as ethanol promote both effects [129].

A birth after oocyte activation by treatment with the calcium ionophore A23187 and ICSI has been obtained in 1994 [130]. Human oocytes injected with round-headed sperm are activated following combination of calcium chloride injection and ionophore treatment. This activation is followed by an apparently normal completion of meiosis, male and female pronuclei formation, embryonic development and successful delivery of a healthy infant [53]. A combination of calcium ionophore A23187 with puromycin stimulates the unfertilized oocytes 20–68 h after ICSI. It results in an activation rate of 91.2% (31/34), a cleavage rate of 64.7% (22/34) and high-quality embryo rate of 44.1% (15/34). Nearly all activated embryos derived from 2PN/2PB had a normal set of sex chromosomes and developed normally [131]. Although calcium ionophore A23187 and puromycin do not appear to be cytotoxic to oocytes and result in pregnancies and the birth of healthy babies when low concentrations are used, the possible teratogenic and mutagenic activity of calcium ionophore A23187 and puromycin needs further investigation in animal models and in humans.

Treatment with 10 mM strontium chloride for 60 min, approximately 30 min after ICSI results in activation and fertilization of all injected oocytes [132], development of the embryos to the blastocyst stage and delivery in patients with repeated fertilization failure [133]. Physical and mental development of the children from birth to 12 months is normal [132]. However, further studies are required to substantiate the finding that strontium chloride treatment is an effective method of artificial oocyte activation.

An electrical field can generate micropores in the cell membrane of gametes and somatic cells to induce sufficient calcium influx through the pores to activate cytoplasm through calcium dependent mechanisms [134]. Mouse oocytes injected with secondary spermatocytes or spermatids are fertilized when stimulated by electroporation and developed into normal offspring when the resultant embryos are transferred to a recipient

[135]. Clinical pregnancy and delivery after oocyte activation by electrostimulation in combination with ICSI in previously failed to fertilize oocytes has been obtained [80]. Electrical stimulation rescues human oocytes that failed to fertilize after ICSI and stimulates them to complete the second meiotic division, to form pronuclei and to undergo early embryonic development [136]. Although the fertilization rate issimilar regardless of the number of electrical pulses applied, subsequent embryo development is dramatically improved in those oocytes that received three electrical pulses [136]. The embryo formation rate in the electrically activated group is 80% compared to 16% in the control group [137]. Although the fertilization rate is significantly higher in the electroactivated group (68%) as compared with that of the control (60%), a higher miscarriage rate is reported in the electroactivated group (5 of 15 pregnancies) compared to the control (3 of 33) [6]. Like any other new assisted reproductive procedure, the impact of electrical activation on oocyte and embryo health must be evaluated in larger studies before this procedure can be considered for routine clinical purposes. Ideally, karyotyping or fluorescent *in situ* hybridization analysis should be performed to assess the incidences of aneuploidy and mosaicism in the resultant embryos.

13. Poor ovarian response

The definition of 'poor response' in the literature is often based on a combination of factors, including the number of mature follicles, the number of oocytes retrieved and the peak estradiol level [138]. The cut-off levels for the number of follicles or oocytes that define poor response vary widely from study to study. Some authors feel that the definition of poor response should also include the degree of ovarian stimulation used and that a low oocyte number is detrimental only when high total dose of follicle stimulating hormone (FSH) has been administered [139]. Various endocrine and ultrasonographic markers and dynamic tests to assess ovarian reserve have been evaluated. Such tests include basal FSH on cycle day 3, clomiphene citrate challenge test, inhibin B, oestrogen, anti-Mullerian hormone, antral follicle counts and ovarian volume. The success of each test can be measured against ovarian response or live birth rate per cycle [140]. However, none of these tests has demonstrated a reliable predictive value and for many women poor ovarian response is not discovered until the first IVF cycle.

Poor response to gonadotropin stimulation occurs more often in older women, but may also occur in young women, regardless of the endocrinologic profile [141]. Poor responders have a significantly lower pregnancy rate per retrieval compared to normal to high responders in the same age group [138]. Although it is possible to have normal embryos and pregnancy in younger poor responders, the fertilization rate and quality of embryos in older poor responders are always low and the chance of achieving pregnancy in these patients is low. Poor responders also have an increased cycle cancellation rate due to retrieval of few or no oocytes and/or TFF. One of the major contributing factors for TFF after ICSI is ≤3 MII oocytes retrieved (Esfandiari *et al.*, 2005a). The rate of fertilization failure increases as the number of injected oocytes decreases [142]. There is a higher chance of having no embryos for transfer and significantly lower pregnancy rates when less than five oocytes are retrieved compared to cases with ≥5 oocytes [143]. Limited information is available on IVM of immature oocytes retrieved from poor responders in conventional stimulation IVF/ICSI cycles and IVM is not a viable alternative to cancellation of IVF cycles in such patients [10].

Fecundity significantly decreases with increasing maternal age [144]. In a classic study of the Hutterite women, sterility increased from just over 10% at 34 years old to over 85% by the age of 44 years [145]. In women, all germ cells are formed during fetal life. The population of germ cells appears to rise steadily from 600 000 at 2 months post conception, reaching a peak of 6 800 000 at 5 months. By the time of birth, the number declines to 2 000 000 of which 50% are atretic. Of the 1 000 000 normal oocytes in the newborn infant, only 300 000 survive to the age of 7 years [146]. Continuous loss of oocytes occurs through the physiological process of follicular growth and atresia throughout life [147].

The incidence of TFF increases with age [10]. Older women are more likely to undergo multiple cycles, have decreased number of oocytes retrieved and a lower number of embryos transferred [9].

14. Oocyte maturity

One of the major causes of TFF after ICSI is a low number of retrieved MII oocytes [10]. About 20% of retrieved oocytes from controlled ovarian stimulation cycles are immature, either at metaphase-I (MI) or germinal-vesicle (GV) stage in human IVF [35]. Some of these oocytes may extrude the first polar body during *in vitro* culture and can be injected in ICSI cycles. This may be a useful strategy for patients with low number of retrieved oocytes. However, embryos derived from immature oocytes do not efficiently translate into pregnancies and live births. Therefore, the clinical significance of using immature oocytes in stimulated cycles needs further investigation [148].

The injection of MI oocytes immediately after denudation results in a high degeneration rate due to increased fragility of the oolemma. The fertilization rate of retrieved MI oocytes that remained MI at the time of ICSI is lower than the fertilization rate of sibling retrieved MI progressing to MII *in vitro* (25% compared to 62.2%, respectively). It is less than half when compared to the fertilization rate of retrieved sibling MII oocytes (69.5%). A high rate of multinucleated oocytes is also found in fertilized MI oocytes injected immediately after denudation [148].

In cases of poor responders and in patients with an unsynchronized cohort of follicles, where the presence of immature oocytes is frequent after stimulation [149], the use of immature oocytes is important in order to increase the number of embryos obtained in each cycle. Based on the assumption that oocyte maturity is a pre-requisite for obtaining normal fertilization, attempts have been made to mature GV and MI oocytes *in vitro* [147]. Despite the use of varying culture techniques and different stimulation protocols, such IVM oocytes consistently have lower fertilization rates, frequent cleavage blocks and overall retarded cleavage rate compared with sibling MII oocytes [147, 150]. The limited number of transfer cycles makes it difficult to draw solid conclusions about the value of transferring these embryos. It should be noted that the immature oocytes collected in stimulated cycles have already been under stimulation with high doses of gonadotropins and are exposed to hCG before retrieval. The nuclear maturation, cytoplasmic maturation and ensuing developmental capacity of these oocytes may very well be different in comparison with immature oocytes collected from small antral follicles of unstimulated ovaries in the typical IVM procedure [151].

15. Oocyte morphology

Poor oocyte morphology is a major determinant of failed or impaired fertilization. Normal features of a healthy mature oocyte at Metaphase-II (MII) include presence of a polar body, a round even shape, light colour cytoplasm with homogenous granularity, a small perivitelline space without debris and a colourless zona pellucida. In denuded oocytes, it is possible to assess the morphology and the nuclear maturity but not the cytoplasmic maturity. The MII oocytes with apparently normal cytoplasmic organization may exhibit extra-cytoplasmic characteristics, such as increased perivitelline space, perivitelline debris and/or fragmentation of the first polar body, which may reduce developmental competence of the oocyte [152]. It is common that extra-cytoplasmic and cytoplasmic dysmorphism occur together in the same oocyte **(Figure 4 and 5)**. The dysmorphic phenotypes, which arise early in meiotic maturation, may be associated with failed fertilization and aneuploidy, while those occurring later in maturation may cause a higher incidence of developmental failure [153, 154].

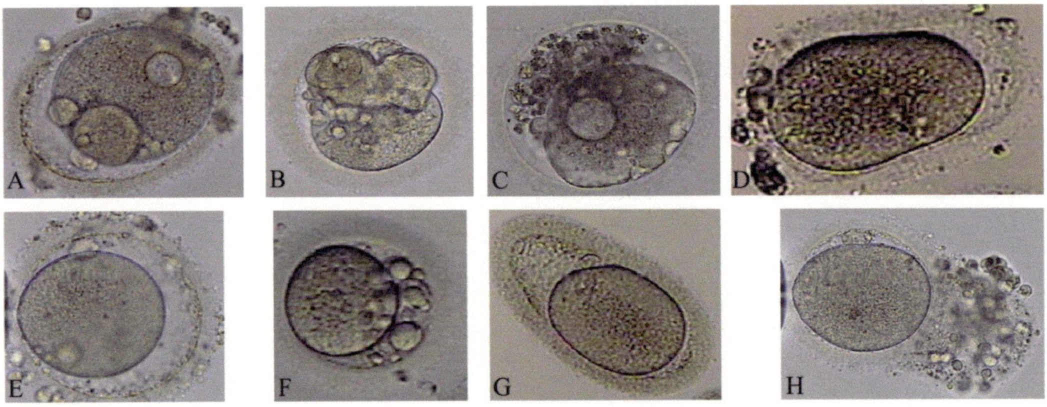

Figure 4. Oocytes in both rows show extra-cytoplasmic and cytoplasmic dysmorphism.

Decreased fertilization rates due to some oocyte dysmorphisms have been reported [152], while others failed to observe that association [155, 156, 157, 158, 159]. Lower pregnancy and implantation rates result when the transferred embryos originate from cycles with >50% dysmorphic oocytes and the same dysmorphism repeats from cycle to cycle [155]. The repetitive organelle clustering is associated with an underlying adverse factor affecting the entire follicular cohort. The presence of a dark cytoplasm decreases by 83% the likelihood of obtaining good quality embryos [160]. However, another study did not find any adverse impact of dark colour of the oocytes on fertilization, embryo development and pregnancy rate [161]. In human oocytes, the cytoplasmic granularity can be homogeneous affecting the whole cytoplasm, or concentrated in the centre with a clear peripheral ring giving a darkened appearance to the cytoplasm [162]. The abnormal changes in the cytoplasm of MII oocytes may be a reflection of delayed cytoplasmic maturation that is unsynchronized with nuclear maturity [163].

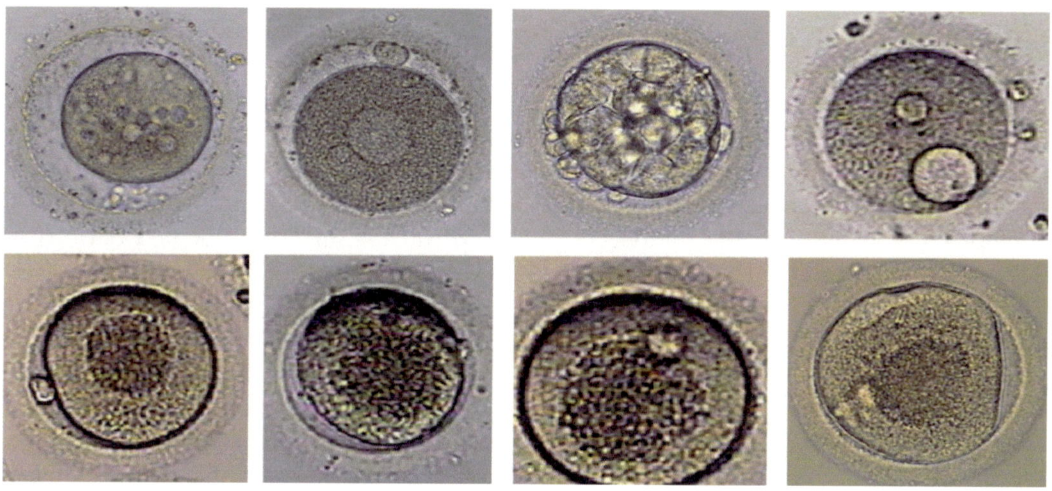

Figure 5. Oocytes in first row represent different degrees of vacuoles in cytoplasm. Each oocytes in second row has increased central granularity.

Normal fertilization, embryo development and live birth are possible after ICSI in oocytes with thick zonae, abnormal morphology or repeated polyspermia following conventional IVF. The oocytes with extreme morphological abnormalities should not be discarded as ICSI can result in fertilization, cleavage and normal embryonic development [164, 161]. The zona-free oocytes may be fertilized normally after ICSI and develop to the blastocyst stage [165]. Pregnancy in human [166] and live birth in mouse [167] and pig [168] have been obtained after transfer of embryos resulting from zona-free oocytes.

16. ICSI after previous ICSI cycle failure

Repeated ICSI treatment can be useful or necessary because there is a high possibility of achieving normal fertilization if a reasonable number of oocytes with normal morphology are available and motile sperm can be found. If there are no motile sperm present in the first ejaculate, a second sample should be required followed by PESA or TESE to obtain motile sperm. In this way, a sufficient number of motile sperm for ICSI are usually found in most men with severe asthenozoospermia.

A history of failed fertilization may be related to some gamete abnormality that may be modified or corrected at the next cycle. It has been documented that for a particular patient, fertilization results can be quite varied when followed through several ICSI cycles at the same centre [169]. The differences between fertilization rates are unexplained, although fluctuations in the gamete quality are probably contributory. Pretreatment endocrine assays and semen analyses prove to be of little value in forecasting failed fertilization. One-third of the patients with TFF achieved pregnancy with their own oocytes in a subsequent ICSI cycle [10]. Since follow-up ICSI treatment has been shown to result in fertilization in 85% of cases, repeated ICSI attempts are suggested in TFF [4, 170].

17. Options for patients after repeated ICSI cycle failure

Physicians should counsel patients based on the best possible evidence available and allow the couple to make an informed choice. The adverse result of a failed ICSI cycle does not imply a hopeless prognosis for future ICSI treatment. Very subtle improvements in semen parameters and/or oocyte yield/quality may result in fertilization in a subsequent ICSI attempt [169]. Otherwise, the options of donor sperm insemination, donated oocytes or embryos, adoption and remaining childless should be discussed with the couple [171].

18. Conclusion

Significant advances have been made in achieving fertilization, pregnancy and live birth in cases with severe male factor infertility, oocyte activation failure and ICSI technique. Usually fertilization is 80-100 percent in mature eggs, however, low or no fertilization can still occur. Most cases of no fertilization occur due to very low number of mature oocytes, failure of oocyte activation or non-availability of appropriate sperm. Repeated ICSI attempts results in fertilization in 85% of cases.

Author details

Murid Javed* and Essam Michael
Astra Fertility Centre, Mississauga, Ontario, Canada

19. References

[1] Benavida CA, Julsen H, Siano L et al. 1999. Intracytoplasmic sperm injection overcomes previous fertilization failure with convention in vitro fertilization. Fertil Steril 72, 1041–1044.
[2] Palermo GD, Neri QV, Takeuchi T et al. 2009. ICSI: where we have been and where we are going. Sem Reprod Med 27,191-201.
[3] Mahutte NG, Arici A 2003. Failed fertilization: is it predictable? Curr Opin Obstet Gynecol 15, 211–218.
[4] Flaherty SP, Payne D, Matthews CD 1998. Fertilization failures and abnormal fertilization after intracytoplasmic sperm injection. Hum Reprod 13, 155-164.
[5] Ebner T, Moser M, Sommergruber M et al. 2004. Complete oocyte activation failure after ICSI can be overcome by a modified injection technique. Hum Reprod 19, 1837–1841.

* Corresponding Author

[6] Mansour R, Fahmy I, Tawab NA et al. 2009. Electrical activation of oocytes after intracytoplasmic sperm injection: a controlled randomized study. Fertil Steril 91, 133-139.

[7] Tesarik J, Rienzi L, Ubaldi F et al. 2002. Use of a modified intracytoplasmic sperm injection technique to overcome sperm-borne and oocyte-borne oocyte activation failures. Fertil Steril 78, 619-24.

[8] Palermo GD, Cohen J, Alikani M et al. 1995. Intracytoplasmic sperm injection: a novel treatment for all forms of male factor infertility. Fertil Steril 63, 1231–1240.

[9] Shen S, Khabani A, Klein N et al. 2003. Statistical analysis of factors affecting fertilization rates and clinical outcome associated with intracytoplasmic sperm injection. Fertil Steril 79, 355–360.

[10] Esfandiari N, Javed MH, Gotlieb L et al. 2005. Complete failed fertilization after intracytoplasmic sperm injection – Analysis of 10 years data. Int J Fertil Women's Med 50, 187-192.

[11] Wang WH, Meng L, Hackett RJ et al. 2001. The spindle observation and its relationship with fertilization after ICSI in living human oocytes. Fertil Steril 75, 348–353.

[12] Wang WH, Meng L, Hackett RJ et al. 2001. Development ability of human oocytes with or without birefringent spindles imaged by Polscope before insemination. Hum Reprod 16, 1464–1468.

[13] Woodward BJ, Montgomery SJ, Hartshorne GM et al. 2008 Spindle position assessment prior to ICSI does not benefit fertilization or early embryo quality. Reprod BioMed Online16, 232-238.

[14] Vanderzwalmen P, Bertin G, Lejeune B et al. 1996 Two essential steps for a successful intracytoplasmic sperm injection: injection of immobilized spermatozoa after rupture of the oolema. Hum Reprod 1l, 540-547.

[15] Ranganathan S, Ganguly AK, Datta K. 1994. Evidence for presence of hyaluronan binding protein on spermatozoa and its possible involvement in sperm function. Mol Reprod Dev. 38(1):69-76.

[16] Yagci A, Murk W, Stronk J, Huszar G. 2010. Spermatozoa bound to solid state hyaluronic acid show chromatin structure with high DNA chain integrity: an acridine orange fluorescence study. J Androl. 31(6):566-72. Epub 2010 Feb 4.

[17] Huszar G, Jakab A, Sakkas D, Ozenci CC, Cayli S, Delpiano E, Ozkavukcu S. 2007. Fertility testing and ICSI sperm selection by hyaluronic acid binding: clinical and genetic aspects. Reprod Biomed Online. 2007 May;14(5):650-63. Review.

[18] Bartoov B, Berkovitz A, Eltes F, Kogosowski A, Menezo Y, Barak Y. 2002. Real-time fine morphology of motile human sperm cells is associated with IVF-ICSI outcome. J Androl23, 1–8.

[19] Balaban B, Yakin K, Alatas C, Oktem O, Isiklar A, Urman B. 2011. Clinical outcome of intracytoplasmic injection of spermatozoa morphologically selected under high magnification: a prospective randomized study. Reprod Biomed Online. Feb 15. [Epub ahead of print]

[20] Vanderzwalmen P, Fallet C. 2010. IMSI: indications, results and reflexions. J Gynecol Obstet Biol Reprod (Paris). 39(1 Suppl):22-5. French.

[21] Mauri AL, Petersen CG, Oliveire JB, Massaro FC, Baruffi LR, Franco JG Jr. 2010. Comparison of day 2 embryo quality after conventional ICSI versus intracytoplasmic morphologically selected sperm injection (IMSI) using sibling oocytes. Eur J Obstet Gynecol Reprod Biol 150:42–46.
[22] Antinori M, Licata E, Dani G, Cerusico F, Versaci C, D'angelo D, Antinori S. 2008. Intracytoplasmic morphologically selected sperm injection: a prospective randomized trial. Reprod Biomed Online 16:835–841.
[23] Knez K, Zorn B, Tomazevic T, Vrtacnik-Bokal E, Virant-Klun I. 2011. The IMSI procedure improves poor embryo development in the same infertile couples with poor semen quality: a comparative prospective randomized study. Reprod Biol Endocrinol. 29;9:123.
[24] Sermondade N, Hafhouf E, Dupont C, Bechoua S, Palacios C, Eustache F, Poncelet C, Benzacken B, Lévy R, Sifer C. 2011. Successful childbirth after intracytoplasmic morphologically selected sperm injection without assisted oocyte activation in a patient with globozoospermia. Hum Reprod. 26(11):2944-9. Epub 2011 Aug 19.
[25] Oliveira JB, Cavagna M, Petersen CG, Mauri AL, Massaro FC, Silva LF, Baruffi RL, Franco JG Jr. 2011. Pregnancy outcomes in women with repeated implantation failures after intracytoplasmic morphologically selected sperm injection (IMSI). Reprod Biol Endocrinol. 22;9:99.
[26] Keefe D, Liu L, Wang W, Silva C. 2003. Imaging meiotic spindles by polarization light microscopy; principles and applications to IVF. Reprod Biomed Online. 7(1):24-9. Review.
[27] Korkmaz C, Cinar O, Akyol M. 2011. The relationship between meiotic spindle imaging and outcome of intracytoplasmic sperm injection: a retrospective study. Gynecol Endocrinol. 27(10):737-41. Epub 2010 Sep 9.
[28] Coticchio G, Sciajno R, Hutt K, Bromfield J, Borini A, Albertini DF. 2010. Comparative analysis of the metaphase II spindle of human oocytes through polarized light and high-performance confocal microscopy. Fertil Steril. 93(6):2056-64. Epub 2009 Feb 24.
[29] De Vos A, Van de Velde H, Joris H, Van Steirteghem A. 1999. In-vitro matured metaphase-I oocytes have a lower fertilization rate but similar embryo quality as mature metaphase-II oocytes after intracytoplasmic sperm injection. Hum Reprod. 14:1859–1863.
[30] Strassburger D, Friedler S, Raziel A, Kasterstein E, Schachter M, Ron-El R. The outcome of ICSI of immature MI oocytes and rescued in vitro matured MII oocytes. Hum Reprod 2004;19:1587–1590.
[31] Eppig JJ, Schultz RM, O'Brien Mand Chesnel, M. 1994. Relationship between the developmental programs controlling nuclear and cytoplasmic maturation of mouse oocytes. Develop Biol. Vol 164 (1) 1–9.
[32] Sundstromand P, Nilsson BO. 1988. Meiotic and cytoplasmic maturation of oocytes collected in stimulated cycles is asynchronous. Hum Reprod Vol 3 (5) 613–619
[33] Balakier H, Sojecki A, Motamedi G, Librach C 2004. Time dependent capability of human oocytes for activation and pronuclear formation during metaphase II arrest," Hum Reprod. Vol 19(4) 982–987
[34] Falcone P, Gambera L, Pisoni M, Lofiego V, De Leo V, Mencaglia L, Piomboni P. 2008. Correlation between oocyte preincubation time and pregnancy rate after intracytoplasmic sperm injection. Gynecol Endocrinol. 24(6):295-9.

[35] Rienzi L, Ubaldi F, Anniballo R, Cerulo G, Greco E. 1998. Preincubation of human oocytes may improve fertilization and embryo quality after intracytoplasmic sperm injection. Hum Reprod 13(4):1014–1019.

[36] Ho JY,Chen MJ,Yi YC, Guu HF, Ho ES. 2003. The effect of preincubation period of oocytes on nuclear maturity, fertilization rate, embryo quality,and pregnancy outcome in IVFandICSI1," J Assist Reprod Genet. Vol 20 (9) 358–364

[37] Isiklar A,Mercan R, Balaban B, Alatas C, Aksoy S, Urman B. 2004. Impact of oocyte pre-incubation time on fertilization, embryo quality and pregnancy rate after intracy toplasmic sperm injection. Reprod BioMed Online. 8 (6) 682–686

[38] Yanagida K, Yazawa H, Katayose H, Suzuki K, Hoshi K, Sato A. 1998. Influence of oocyte preincubation time on fertilization after intracytoplasmic sperm injection. Hum Reprod Vol 13 (8) 2223–2226.

[39] Malgorzata K, Depa-Martynów M, Butowska W et al. 2007 Human spermatozoa ultrastructure assessment in the infertility treatment by assisted reproduction technique. Arch Androl 53, 297-302.

[40] Francavilla S, Cordeschi G, Pelliccione F et al. 2007 Isolated teratozoospermia: a cause of male sterility in the era of ICSI? Front Biosci 12, 69-88.

[41] Kupker W, Schulze W, Diedrich K 1998 Ultrastructure of gametes and intracytoplasmic sperm injection. The significance of sperm morphology. Hum Reprod 13 (Suppl. 1), 99–106.

[42] Yu JJ, Xu YM 2004 Ultrastructural defects of acrosome in infertile men. Arch Androl 50, 405–409.

[43] Lamb DJ 1999 Debate: Is ICSI a Genetic Bomb? Yes. J Androl20, 23–33.

[44] Zhang S, Wang N, He B, Cheng J, Xi S, Wang SM, Gao Y, Wang J. 2012. Sperm head vacuoles-light microscopic and ultrastructural observations: a case report. Ultrastruct Pathol. 36(3):185-8.

[45] Perdrix A, Saïdi R, Ménard JF, Gruel E, Milazzo JP, Macé B, Rives N. 2012. Relationship between conventional sperm parameters and motile sperm organelle morphology examination (MSOME). Int J Androl. Mar 15. doi: 10.1111/j.1365-2605.2012.01249.x. [Epub ahead of print]

[46] Cassuto NG, Hazout A, Hammoud I, Balet R, Bouret D, Barak Y, Jellad S, Plouchart JM, Selva J, Yazbeck C. 2012. Correlation between DNA defect and sperm-head morphology. Reprod Biomed Online. 24(2):211-8. Epub 2011 Oct 22.

[47] Guthauser B, Albert M, Ferfouri F, Ray PF, Rabiey G, Selva J, Vialard F. 2011. Inverse correlation between chromatin condensation and sperm head size in a case of enlarged sperm heads. Reprod Biomed Online. 23(6):711-6. Epub 2011 Jul 22.

[48] Dam AH, Feenstra I, Westphal JR et al. 2007 Globozoospermia revisited. Hum Reprod Update 13, 63-75.

[49] Kullander S, Rausing A 1975. On round-headed human spermatozoa. International Journal of Fertility 20, 33-40.

[50] Kilani Z, Ismail R, Ghunaim S et al. 2004 Evaluation and treatment of familial globozoospermia in five brothers. Fertil steril 82, 1436-1439.

[51] Wan L, An LM, Xia XY. 2011. Molecular genetics of globozoospermia: an update. Zhonghua Nan Ke Xue. 17(10):935-8. Review. Chinese.

[52] Battaglia DE, Koehler JK, Klein NA et al. 1997 Failure of oocyte activation after intracytoplasmic sperm injection using round-headed sperm. Fertil steril 68, 118-122.

[53] Rybouchkin AV, Van der Straeten F, Quatacker J et al. 1997 Fertilization and pregnancy after assisted oocyte activation and intracytoplasmic sperm injection in a case of round-headed sperm associated with deficient oocyte activation capacity. Fertil steril 68, 1144-1147.

[54] Stone S, O'Mahony F, Khalaf Y et al. 2000 A normal live birth after intracytoplasmic sperm injection for globozoospermia without assisted oocyte activation. Hum Reprod 15, 139–141.

[55] Edirisinghe WR, Murch AR, Junk SM et al. 1998 Cytogenetic analysis of unfertilized oocytes following intracytoplasmic sperm injection using spermatozoa from a globozoospermic man. Hum Reprod 13, 3094–3098.

[56] Aitken RJ, De Iuliis GN 2007 Origins and consequences of DNA damage in male germ cells. Reprod BioMed Online 14, 727-733.

[57] Virro MR, Larson-Cook KL, Evenson DP 2004 Sperm chromatin structure assay (SCSA) parameters are related to fertilization, blastocyst development, and ongoing pregnancy in in vitro fertilization and intracytoplasmic sperm injection cycles. Fertil steril 81, 1289–1295.

[58] Braude P, Bolton V, Moore S 1988 Human gene expression first occurs between the four- and eight-cell stages of preimplantation development. Nature 332, 459–461.

[59] Twigg JP, Irvine DS, Aitken RJ 1998 Oxidative damage to DNA in human spermatozoa does not preclude pronucleus formation at intracytoplasmic sperm injection. Hum Reprod 13, 1864–1871.

[60] Tesarik J, Greco E, Mendoza C 2004 Late, but not early, paternal effect on human embryo development is related to sperm DNA fragmentation. Hum Reprod 19, 611–615.

[61] Sun JG, Jurisicova A, Casper RF 1997 Detection of deoxyribonucleic acid fragmentation in human sperm: correlation with fertilization in vitro. Biol Reprod 56, 602-607.

[62] Irvine DS, Twigg JP, Gordon EL et al. 2001 DNA integrity in human spermatozoa: relationships with semen quality. J Androl21, 33–44.

[63] Lopes S, Jurisicova A, Casper RF 1998 Gamete-specific DNA fragmentation in unfertilized human oocytes after intracytoplasmic sperm injection. Hum Reprod 13, 703-708.

[64] Sikora J, Kempisty B, Jedrzejczak P et al. 2006 Influence of DNA damage on fertilizing capacity of spermatozoa. Przeglad lekarski 63, 800-802.

[65] Moskovtsev S, Alladin N, Lo K, Jarvi K, Mullen J, Librach C. 2012. A comparison of ejaculated and testicular spermatozoa aneuploidy rates in patients with high sperm DNA damage. Syst Biol Reprod Med. 2012 Mar 20. [Epub ahead of print]

[66] Evenson DP, Larson KL, Jost LK 2002 Sperm chromatin structure assay: its clinical use for detecting sperm DNA fragmentation in male infertility and comparisons with other techniques. J Androl23, 25–43.

[67] Potts RJ, Newbury CJ, Smith G et al. 1999 Sperm chromatin changes associated with male smoking. Mutation Research 423, 103–11.

[68] Bungum M, Humaidan P, Axmon A et al. 2007 Sperm DNA integrity assessment in prediction of assisted reproduction technology outcome. Hum Reprod 22, 174-179.

[69] Spano M, Seli E, Bizzaro D et al. 2005 The significance of sperm nuclear DNA strand breaks on reproductive outcome. Current Opinion in Obstetrics & Gynecology 17, 255-260.
[70] Aitken RJ, De Iuliis GN, McLachlan RI 2009 Biological and clinical significance of DNA damage in the male germ line. Int J Androl 32, 46-56.
[71] Beshay VE, Bukulmez O. 2012. Sperm DNA damage: how relevant is it clinically? Curr Opin Obstet Gynecol 24(3):172-9.
[72] Saremi A, Esfandiari N, Salehi N et al. 2002 The first successful pregnancy following injection of testicular round spermatid in Iran. Archiv Androl48, 315-319.
[73] Jurisicova A, Lopes S, Meriano J et al. 1999 DNA damage in round spermatids of mice with targeted disruption of PP1c gamma gene and in testicular biopsies of patients with non-destructive azoospermia. Mol Hum Reprod 5, 323-330.
[74] Zech H, Vanderzwalmen P, Prapas Y et al. 2000 Congenital malformations after intracytoplasmic injection of spermatids. Hum Reprod 15, 969 –971.
[75] The Practice Committee of American Society for Reproductive Medicine, Practice Committee of Society for Assisted Reproductive Technology 2008 Round spermatid nucleus injection (ROSNI). Fertil steril 90 (Supp l), S199-201.
[76] Johnson RT, Rao PN 1970 Mammalian cell fusion: induction of premature chromosome condensation in interphase nuclei. Nature 226, 717–722.
[77] Schmiady H, Sperling K, Kentenich H et al. 1986 Prematurely condensed human sperm chromosomes after in vitro fertilization (IVF). Human Genetics 74, 441–443.
[78] Ma S, Kalousek DK, Yuen BH 1994 Chromosome investigation in in vitro fertilization failure. J Assist Reprod Gen1,445–451.
[79] Van Blerkom J, Davis PW, Merriam J 1994 Fertilization and early embryology: a retrospective analysis of unfertilized and presumed parthenogenetically activated human oocytes demonstrates a high frequency of sperm penetration. Hum Reprod 9, 2381–2388.
[80] Yanagida K, Katayose H, Yazawa H et al. 1999 Successful fertilization and pregnancy following ICSI and electrical oocyte activation. Hum Reprod 14, 1307-1311.
[81] Grasa P, Coward K, Young C et al. 2008 The pattern of localization of the putative oocyte activation factor, phospholipase Cz, in uncapacitated, capacitated, and ionophore-treated human spermatozoa. Hum Reprod 23, 2513–2522.
[82] Balhorn R 1982. A model for the structure of chromatin in mammalian sperm. The Journal of Cell Biology 93, 298–305.
[83] Dozortsev D, Qian C, Ermilov A et al. 1997 Sperm-associated oocyte-activating factor is released from the spermatozoon within 30 minutes after injection as a result of the sperm–oocyte interaction. Hum Reprod 12, 2792-2796.
[84] Ma S, Yuen BH 2001 Intracytoplasmic sperm injection could minimize the incidence of prematurely condensed human sperm chromosomes. Fertil Steril 75, 1095–1101.
[85] Calafell JM, Badenas J, Egozcue J et al. 1991 Premature chromosome condensation as a sign of oocyte immaturity. Hum Reprod 6, 1017–1021.
[86] Rosenbuch BE 2000 Frequency and patterns of premature sperm chromosome condensation in oocytes failing to fertilize after intracytoplasmic sperm injection. J Assist Reprod Gen17, 253–259.

[87] Schmiady H, Schulze W, Scheiber I et al. 2005 High rate of premature chromosome condensation in human oocytes following microinjection with round-headed sperm: Case report. Hum Reprod 20, 1319–1323.
[88] Nasr-Esfahani MH, Razavi S, Tavalaee M 2008 Failed fertilization after ICSI and spermiogenic defects. Fertil Steril 89, 892-898.
[89] Chemes H, Alvarez Sedo C. 2012. Tales of the tail and sperm head aches: changing concepts on the prognostic significance of sperm pathologies affecting the head, neck and tail. Asian J Androl. 14(1):14-23. doi: 10.1038/aja.2011.168. Epub 2011 Dec 26.
[90] Konc J, Kanyo K, Cseh S 2006 Deliveries from embryos fertilized with spermatozoa obtained from cryopreserved testicular tissue. J Assist Reprod Gen23, 247–252.
[91] Wang CW, Lai YM, Wang ML et al. 1997 Pregnancy after intracytoplasmic injection of immotile sperm. A case report. J Reprod Med42, 448-450.
[92] Kusakabe H, Szczygiel MA, Whittingham DG et al. 2001 Maintenance of genetic integrity in frozen and freeze-dried mouse spermatozoa. Proceedings of the National Academy of Sciences of the United States of America 98, 13501–13506.
[93] Ghosh S, Chattopadhyay R, Bose G, Ganesh A, Das S, Chakravarty BN. 2012. Selection of birefringent spermatozoa under Polscope: effect on intracytoplasmic sperm injection outcome. Andrologia. Feb 28. doi: 10.1111/j.1439-0272.2011.01258.x. [Epub ahead of print]
[94] Sallam H, Farrag A, Agameya A, El-Garem Y, Ezzeldin F. 2005. The use of the modified hypo-osmotic swelling test for the selection of immotile testicular spermatozoa in patients treated with ICSI: a randomized controlled study. Hum Reprod 2005; 20: 3435–40.
[95] Gerber P, Kruse R, Hirchenhain J, Kru¨ ssel J, Neumann N. 2008. Pregnancy after laser assisted selection of viable spermatozoa before intracytoplasmatic sperm injection in a couple with male primary cilia dyskinesia. Fertil Steril 2008; 89: 1826.e9–12.
[96] Kordus R, Price R, Davis J, Whitman-Elia G. Successful twin birth following blastocyst culture of embryos derived from the immotile ejaculated spermatozoa from a patient with primary ciliary dyskinesia: a case report. J Assist Reprod Genet 2008; 25: 437–43.
[97] Mangoli V, Mangoli R, Dandekar S, Suri K, Desai S. Selection of viable spermatozoa from testicular biopsies: a comparative study between pentoxifylline and hypoosmotic swelling test. Fertil Steril 2011; 95: 631–4.
[98] Hattori H, Nakajo Y, Ito C, Toyama Y, Toshimori K, Kyono K. 2011. Birth of a healthy infant after intracytoplasmic sperm injection using pentoxifylline-activated sperm from a patient with Kartagener's syndrome. Fertil Steril. 95(7):2431.e9-11. Epub 2011 Apr 20.
[99] Jeyendran RS, Van der Ven HH, Perez-Pelaez M et al. 1984 Development of an assay to assess the functional integrity of the human sperm membrane and its relationship to other semen characteristics. J Reprod Fertil 70, 219-228.
[100] Casper RF, Meriano JS, Jarvi KA et al. 1996 The hypo-osmotic swelling test for selection of viable sperm for intracytoplasmic sperm injection in men with complete asthenozoospermia. Fertil Steril 65, 972-976.
[101] Liu V, Tsai YL, Katz E et al. 1997 High fertilization rate obtained after intracytoplasmic sperm injection with 100% nonmotile spermatozoa selected by using a simple modified hypo-osmotic swelling test. Fertil Steril 68, 373-375.

[102] Ahmadi A, Ng SC 1997 The single sperm curling test, a modified hypo-osmotic swelling test, as a potential technique for the selection of viable sperm for intracytoplasmic sperm injection. Fertil Steril 68, 346-350.

[103] Verheyen G, Joris H, Crits K et al. 1997 Comparison of different hypo-osmotic swelling solutions to select viable immotile spermatozoa for potential use in intracytoplasmic sperm injection. Hum Reprod Update 3, 195-203.

[104] Sallam HN, Farrag A, Agameya AF et al. 2001 The use of a modified hypo-osmotic swelling test for the selection of viable ejaculated and testicular immotile spermatozoa in ICSI. Hum Reprod 16, 272-276.

[105] Yildirim G, Ficicioglu C, Akcin O, Attar R, Tecellioglu N, Yencilek F (2009). Can pentoxifylline improve the sperm motion and ICSI success in the primary ciliary dyskinesia? Arch Gynecol Obstet. 279(2):213-5. Epub 2008 May 7.

[106] Palermo GD, Joris H, Devroey P et al. 1992 Pregnancies after intracytoplasmic injection of single spermatozoon into an oocyte. Lancet 340, 17–18.

[107] Proctor M, Johnson N, Van Peperstraten AM et al. 2009 Techniques for surgical retrieval of sperm prior to intra-cytoplasmic sperm injection (ICSI) for azoospermia. Cochrane Database for Systematic Reviews 2, CD002807.

[108] Wennerholm UB, Bergh C, Hamberger L et al. 2000 Obstetric outcome of pregnancies following ICSI, classified according to sperm origin and quality. Hum Reprod 15, 1189–1194.

[109] Bulkumez O, Yucel A, Yarali H et al. 2001 The origin of spermatozoa does not affect intracytoplasmic sperm injection outcome. Eur J Obstet Gyn Reprod Biol94, 250–255.

[110] Silber SJ, Nagy ZP, Liu J 1994 Conventional in-vitro fertilization vs ICSI for patients requiring microsurgical sperm aspiration. Hum Reprod 9, 1705–1709.

[111] Lewis S, Klonoff-Cohen H 2005 What factors affect intracytoplasmic sperm injection outcomes? Obstet & Gynecol Sur 60, 111-123.

[112] Matyas S, Papp G, Kovacs P et al. 2005 Intracytoplasmic injection with motile and immotile frozen-thawed testicular spermatozoa (the Hungarian experience). Andrologia 37, 25–28.

[113] Halliday J. 2012. Outcomes for offspring of men having ICSI for male factor infertility. Asian J Androl. 14(1):116-20. doi: 10.1038/aja.2011.71. Epub 2011 Dec 12.

[114] Yamano S, Nakagawa K, Nakasaka H et al. 2000 Fertility failure and oocyte activation. J Med Invest 47, 1-8.

[115] Miyazaki S, Ito M 2006 Calcium signals for egg activation in mammals. J Pharmacol Sci 100, 545–552.

[116] Swann K 1990 A cytosolic sperm factor stimulates repetitive calcium increases and mimics fertilization in hamster eggs. Development 110, 1295–1302.

[117] Wu H, He CL, Fissore RA 1997 Injection of a porcine sperm factor triggers calcium oscillations in mouse oocytes and bovine eggs. Mol Reprod Develop 46, 176–189.

[118] Jones KT, Cruttwell C, Parrington J, Swann K 1998 A mammalian sperm cytosolic phospholipase C activity generates inositol trisphosphate and causes Ca2+ release in sea urchin egg homogenates. FEBS Letters 437, 297–300.

[119] Wu H, Smyth J, Luzzi V et al. 2001. Sperm factor induces intracellular free calcium oscillations by stimulating the phosphoinositide pathway. Biol Reprod 64, 1338–1349.

[120] Rice A, Parrington J, Jones KT et al. 2000 Mammalian sperm contain a Ca(2+)-sensitive phospholipase C activity that can generate InsP3 from PIP2 associated with intracellular organelles. Develop Biol 228, 125–135.

[121] Saunders CM 2002 PLCζ: a sperm-specific trigger of Ca(2+) oscillations in eggs and embryo development. Development 129, 3533–3544.

[122] Kouchi Z, Fukami K, Shikano T et al. 2004 Recombinant phospholipase Czeta has high Ca2+ sensitivity and induces Ca2+ oscillations in mouse eggs. J Biol Chem 279, 10408–10412.

[123] Kurokawa M, Yoon SY, Alfandari D et al. 2007 Proteolytic processing of phospholipase Czeta and [Ca2+]i oscillations during mammalian fertilization. Develop Biol 312, 407–418.

[124] Yoon SY, Jellerette T, Salicioni AMJ et al. 2008 Human sperm devoid of PLC, zeta 1 fail to induce Ca(2+) release and are unable to initiate the first step of embryo development. The Journal of Clinical Investigation 118, 3671-3681.

[125] Heindryckx B, Van der Elst J, De Sutter P et al. 2005 Treatment option for sperm- or oocyte-related fertilization failure: assisted oocyte activation following diagnostic heterologous ICSI. Hum Reprod 20, 2237–2241.

[126] Vanden MF, Nikiforaki D, De Gheselle S, Dullaerts V, Van den Abbeel E, Gerris J, Heindryckx B, De Sutter P. Assisted oocyte activation is not beneficial for all patients with a suspected oocyte-related activation deficiency. Hum Reprod. 2012 Apr 4. [Epub ahead of print]

[127] Nakada K, Mizuno J 1998 Intracellular calcium responses in bovine oocytes induced by spermatozoa and by reagents. Theriogenology 50, 269–282.

[128] Cuthbertson KSR, Whittingham DG, Cobbold PH 1981. Free Ca2+ increases in exponential phases during mouse oocyte activation. Nature 294, 754–757.

[129] Loi P, Ledda S, Fulka Jr J et al. 1998 Development of parthenogenetic and cloned ovine embryos: effect of activation protocols. Biol Reprod 58, 1177–1187.

[130] Hoshi K, Yanagida K, Yazawa H et al. 1995 Intracytoplasmic sperm injection using immobilized or motile human spermatozoon. Fertil Steril 63, 1241-1245.

[131] Lu Q, Zhao Y, Gao X et al. 2006 Combination of calcium ionophore A23187 with puromycin salvages human unfertilized oocytes after ICSI. Eur J Obstet Gyn Reprod Biol126, 72-76.

[132] Kyono K, Kumagai S, Nishinaka C et al. 2008 Birth and follow-up of babies born following ICSI using $SrCl_2$ oocyte activation. Reprod BioMed Online 17, 53-58.

[133] Yanagida K, Morozumi K, Katayose H et al. 2006 Case report: Successful pregnancy after ICSI with strontium oocyte activation in low rates of fertilization. Reprod BioMed Online 3, 801–806.

[134] Ozil JP 1990 The parthenogenetic development of rabbit oocytes after repetitive pulsatile electrical stimulation. Development 109, 117–127.

[135] Kimura Y, Yanagimachi R 1995 Development of normal mice from oocytes injected with secondary spermatocyte nuclei. Biol Reprod 53, 855–862.

[136] Zhang J, Wang C, Blaszcyzk A et al. 1999 Electrical activation and in vitro development of human oocytes that fail to fertilize after intracytoplasmic sperm injection. Fertil Steril 72, 509-512.
[137] Manipalviratn S, Ahnonkitpanit V, Numchaisrika P et al. 2006 Results of direct current electrical activation of failed-to-fertilize oocytes after intracytoplasmic sperm injection. J Reprod Med51, 493-499.
[138] Saldeen P, Källen K, Sundström P 2007 The probability of successful IVF outcome after poor ovarian response. Acta Obstet Gynecol Scan 86, 457-461.
[139] Kailasam C, Keay SD, Wilson P et al. 2004 Defining poor ovarian response during IVF cycles, in women < 40 years, and its relationship with treatment outcome. Hum Reprod 19, 1544-1547.
[140] Sun W, Stegmann BJ, Henne M et al. 2008 A new approach to ovarian reserve testing. Fertility Sterility 90, 2196-2202.
[141] Lashen H, Ledger W, Lopez-Bernal A et al. 1999 Poor responders to ovulation induction-is proceeding to in-vitro fertilization worthwhile? Hum Reprod 14, 964- 969.
[142] Yanagida K 2004 Complete fertilization failure in ICSI. Human Cell 17, 187-193.
[143] Melie NA, Adeniyi OA, Igbineweka OM et al. 2003 Predictive value of the number of oocytes retrieved at ultrasound-directed follicular aspiration with regard to fertilization rates and pregnancy outcome in intracytoplasmic sperm injection treatment cycles. Fertil Steril 80, 1376–1379.
[144] Devroey P, Godoy H, Smitz J et al. 1996 Female age predicts embryonic implantation after ICSI: a case-controlled study. Hum Reprod 11, 1324–1327.
[145] Tietze C 1957 Reproductive span and rate of reproduction among Hutterite women. Fertil Steril 8, 89–97.
[146] Baker TG 1963 A Quantitative and Cytological Study of Germ Cells in Human Ovaries. Proceedings of the Royal Society of London, Series B, Biological Sciences 158, 417-433.
[147] Djahanbakhch O, Ezzati M, Zosmer A 2007 Reproductive ageing in women. The Journal of Pathology 211, 219-231.
[148] Shu Y, Gebhardt J, Watt J et al. 2007 Fertilization, embryo development, and clinical outcome of immature oocytes from stimulated intracytoplasmic sperm injection cycles. Fertil Steril 87, 1022-1027.
[149] Smitz J, Cortvrindt R 1999 Oocyte in-vitro maturation and follicle culture: current clinical achievements and future directions. Hum Reprod 14, 145-161.
[150] Chen SU, Chen HF, Lien YR et al. 2000 Schedule to inject IVM-MI oocytes may increase pregnancy after intracytoplasmic sperm injection. Archiv Androl 44, 197-205.
[151] Sun QY, Lai L, Bonk A et al. 2001 Cytoplasmic changes in relation to nuclear maturation and early embryo developmental potential of porcine oocytes: effects of gonadotropins, cumulus cells, follicular size, and protein synthesis inhibition. Molecular Reprod Develop 59, 192– 198.
[152] Xia P 1997 Intracytoplasmic sperm injection: correlation of oocyte grade based on polar body, perivitelline space and cytoplasmic inclusions with fertilization rate and embryo quality. Hum Reprod 12, 1750-1755.

[153] Van Blerkom J, Henry G 1992 Oocyte dysmorphism and aneuploidy in meiotically mature oocytes after ovarian stimulation. Hum Reprod 7, 379-390.
[154] Ebner T, Moser M, Tews G 2006 Is oocyte morphology prognostic of embryo developmental potential after ICSI? Reprod BioMed Online 12, 507-512.
[155] Meriano JS, Alexis J, Visram-Zaver S et al. 2001 Tracking of oocyte dysmorphisms for ICSI patients may prove relevant to the outcome in subsequent patient cycles. Hum Reprod 16, 2118-2123.
[156] Mikkelsen AL, Lindenberg S 2001 Morphology of in-vitro matured oocytes: impact on fertility potential and embryo quality. Hum Reprod 16, 17I4-I7I8.
[157] Ciotti PM, Nmarangelo L, Morsclli-Labate AM et al. 2004 First polar body morphology before ICSI is not related to embryo quality or pregnancy rate. Hum Reprod 19, 2334-2339.
[158] Otsuki J, Okada A, Morimoto K et al. 2004 The relationship between pregnancy outcome and smooth endoplasmic reticulum clusters in metaphase II human oocytes. Hum Reprod 19, 1591- 1597.
[159] De Santis L, Cino I, Rabellotti E et al. 2005 Polar body morphology and spindle imaging as predictors of oocyte quality. Reprod BioMed Online 11, 36-42.
[160] Ten J, Mendiola J, Vioque J et al. 2007 Donor oocyte dysmorphisms and their influence on fertilization and embryo quality. Reprod BioMed Online 14, 40-48.
[161] Esfandiari N, Burjaq H, Gotlieb L et al. 2006. Brown oocytes: implications for assisted reproductive technology. Fertil Steril 86, 1522-1525.
[162] Serhal PF, Ranieri DM, Kinis A et al. 1997 Oocyte morphology predicts outcome of intracytoplasmic sperm injection. Hum Reprod 12, 1267-1270.
[163] Katz N, Tur-Kaspa I 2000 Cytoplasmic maturity of metaphase II human oocytes: Biologic importance and clinical implications for in vitro fertilization. Reprod Technol 10, 170-173.
[164] Esfandiari N, Ryan EA, Gotlieb L et al. 2005 Successful pregnancy following transfer of embryos from oocytes with abnormal zona pellucida and cytoplasm morphology. Reprod BioMed Online 11, 620-623.
[165] JelinkovaL, Pavelkova J, Rezabek K et al. 2001 Treatment of infertility using oocytes without the zona pellucida. Ceská gynekologie 65, 456-459.
[166] Stanger JD, Stevenson K, Lakmaker A et al. 2001 Pregnancy following fertilization of zona-free, coronal cell intact human ova: Case Report. Hum Reprod 16, 164-167.
[167] Naito K, Toyoda Y, Yanagimachi R 1992 Production of normal mice from oocytes fertilized and developed without zonae pellucidae. Hum Reprod 7, 281-285.
[168] Wu GM, Lai L, Mao J et al. 2004 Birth of piglets by in vitro fertilization of zona-free porcine oocytes. Theriogenology 62, 1544-1556.
[169] Moomjy M, Sills ES, Rosenwaks Z et al. 1998 Implications of complete fertilization failure after intracytoplasmic sperm injection for subsequent fertilization and reproductive outcome. Hum Reprod 13, 2212–2216.
[170] Rouzi AA, Amarin Z 2002 Repeat intracytoplasmic sperm injection. Clinical perspective. Saudi Med J 23, 1470-1472.
[171] Wen SW, Walker M, Léveillé MC et al. 2004 Intracytoplasmic sperm injection: promises and challenges. Can Med Ass J 171, 845-846.

Chapter 6

SubEndometrial Embryo Delivery (SEED) with Egg Donation – Mechanical Embryo Implantation

Michael Kamrava and Mei Yin

Additional information is available at the end of the chapter

http://dx.doi.org/10.5772/50034

1. Introduction

Egg quality at retrieval in IVF cycles is one of the prime prognostic factors of a successful outcome in IVF cycles. Thus egg donors provide a unique opportunity for assessing the feasibility of new protocols and techniques. In these situations, where the primary reason for resorting to IVF is peri/post menopausal state of the woman, using egg donors assures that at least the quality of the eggs are optimum, and most often the sperm quality, embryo quality at transfer, the recipient's uterus and endometrial condition are not adversely affected.

In patients undergoing *in vitro* fertilization (IVF) procedures one major set of hurdles, which often prevents healthy embryos from resulting in pregnancies, are problems associated with endometrial receptivity and implantation (1-4). From a clinical practice perspective in our new age of pre-implantation diagnosis and screening, the embryo transfer process may now be regarded as a rate limiting factor. Various techniques for embryo transfer (ET) have been advocated to increase pregnancy rates while reducing side effects from the procedure, such as lost embryos and ectopic pregnancies (5-7, 48). In addition, the advantages of using different catheters have been debated (8-11). These methods, however, use a "blind" technique of catheter introduction into the uterus. Since the embryo(s), having the zona pellucida at time of transfer, floats in the uterine cavity between one to three days from the time of transfer, the problems of "lost embryos" and the occurrence of ectopic pregnancies persist. We have hypothesized that the mechanical insertion of the blastocyst into the endometrium under direct visualization would increase the implantation and clinical pregnancy rate of IVF. The aim of this study was to re-investigate the potential of sub-endothelial ET, a procedure which originated from early mouse experiments (10) and in humans in the mid to late 1990's (12, 13) via trans-abdominal approaches. In contrast to these earlier investigations we propose to use hysteroscopy as a less invasive, visually confirmed, precise and reliable technique to direct and effect the implantation procedure.

2. Materials and methods

2.1. Patients

The study was approved by local review board at West Coast IVF Clinic, Inc. and a fully informed consent was obtained from all patients. There were 21 consecutive patients between 34-50 years of age with a diagnosis of peri/postmenopause or premature ovarian failure with or without tubal disease. They underwent 24 fresh IVF cycles in this study. Controlled ovarian hyperstimulation was initiated with follitropin β® (Follistim®, Organon Pharmaceuticals, Inc.). Premature surge of endogenous gonadotropins were controlled with ganirelix acetate (Antagon®, Organon Pharmaceuticals, Inc.). Oocyte retrieval was carried out in an office setting under local anesthesia and mild sedation. Embryo culturing was performed using sequential media (G1 and G2; Vitrolife, or Early Cleavage Medium® supplemented with SSS and Complete Multiblast Medium® with SSS; Irvine Scientific, USA) to day five or six. Up to 2 grade 1 expanded/hatching blastocysts were transferred (Fig 1A). Recipients were down regulated with long acting GnRH analog (Leuprolide acetate Depot, Abbott, USA). The endometrium was primed with Estradiol 2 mg tid until the day of donor egg retrieval, when it was continued or reduced to 1 mg tid. Luteal support was maintained with Progesterone in oil IM 50-100 mg/progesterone vaginal tablets (Endometrin®, Ferring, USA), 100 mg tid. until the day of Pregnancy test. If the test was positive progesterone was continued through the 8th week of pregnancy or sooner until a rise in serum progesterone was noted as the pregnancy progressed.

Serum human chorionic gonadotropin (hCG) was quantified on the tenth or eleventh day after SEED was performed on day six or five after retrieval, respectively. Although the assay sensitivity for detection of hCG was at 2 IU/ml a concentration of >5 IU/ml was used for confirmation of pregnancy.

2.2. Description of hysteroscopic implantation

A lightweight flexible mini- hysteroscope (Storz™) was used for visualization of the endometrial cavity (Fig 1D). The scope incorporates a flexible distal end of 3mm in diameter with a straight through operating channel. In addition, the optic filter is directly connected to a light source, decreasing the weight of the scope. Nitrogen gas instead of CO2 is used for uterine distention. Nitrogen gas is inert and is used in the trimixture of Nitrogen, Oxygen and Carbon Dioxide utilized for embryo culture in an IVF laboratory. Gas pressure is set at max 70 mm mercury (HG). A maximum of 50 cc of gas is used

during the entire procedure. The transfer catheter is polycarbonate based with a tapered tip (to 500 μm), beveled to 45-60° (Initially made by Cook OB/GYN™, Spencer, Indiana, USA and subsequently made by Precision Reproduction, LLC Los Angeles, CA 90212 USA). The catheter is inserted to a distance of 0.5cm horizontally and to a depth of approximately 1mm below the surface of the endometrium, and 2 cm away from the junction of tuboendometrial border as observed hysteroscopically where the endometrium is thickest as seen through the hysteroscope. The embryo(s) is deposited under direct hysteroscopic visualization (Fig 1D) using a 100 μl Hamilton syringe (Hamilton Company; Nevada, USA). No more than 2 embryos were implanted at any one site.

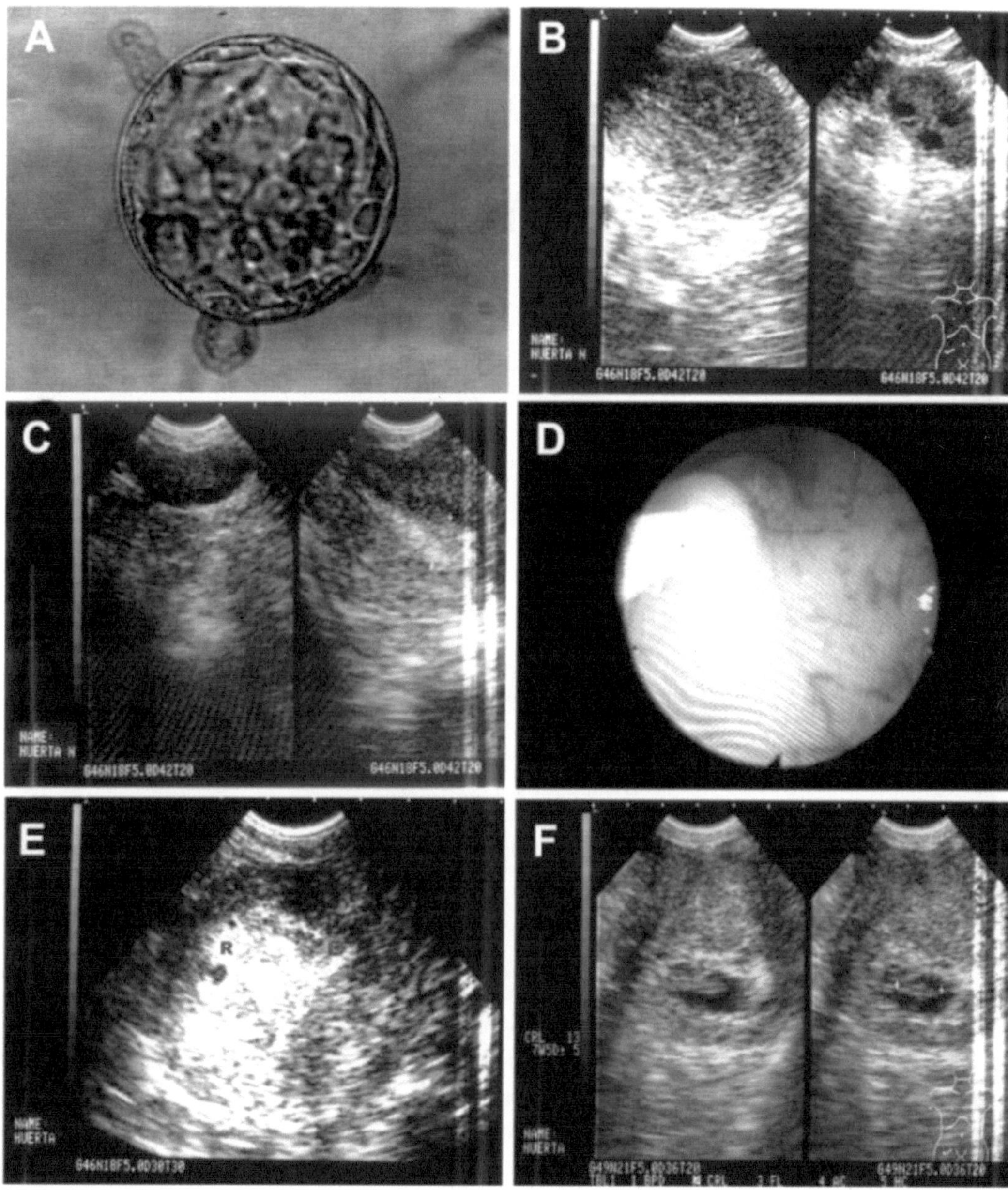

Figure 1. Stages of subendometrial embryo transfer. Expanded hatching blastocyst (A); estrogenic endometrium (B); progestational endometrium (C); subendometrial embryo transfer (D); early gestational sac at 5 weeks (E); fetus at 6 weeks (F).

3. Results

In this series, 24 IVF cycles in 21 patients were completed. Endometrial thicknesses varied between 7 and 16mm by transvaginal ultrasound. There were sixteen positive βhCG's at levels greater than 5 IU/ml. There were five biochemical pregnancies, and eleven clinical pregnancies as evidenced by the presence of a gestational sac (Fig 1E) visualized by ultrasound examination at five weeks of gestation and heart beat at six weeks of gestation (Fig 1F). There were 5 spotaneous abortions. Healthy babies were delivered by seven patients. No ectopic pregnancies (tubal, placenta previa, cervical, or heterotopic) were seen (Table 1). There were 4 twins from day five and none from day 6 implantations.

	Day 5 Implantation	Day 6 Implantation	Combined D5 and D6
Patient starts	14	10	24
Total Pregnancy/Start	8(57%)	8(80%)	16(67%)
Biochemical Pregnancy	2	2	4
Ectopic Pregnancy	**0**	**0**	**0**
Spotaneous Abortions	2	3	5
Multiple Pregnancy	4	0	4
Live/Start	4 (29%)	3 (30%)	**7 (29%)**

Table 1.

4. Discussion

Various techniques and technologies for ET have been proposed since the introduction of IVF. This list includes ultrasound-controlled transcervical intrauterine transfer or transmyometrial transfer and more invasive procedures, often referred to as surgical ET, which include: gamete intra-fallopian transfer (GIFT), zygote intra-fallopian transfer (ZIFT), pronuclear stage transfer and embryo intrafallopian transfer (EIFT) (14-17). Although ultrasound guided ET was desired to improve successful pregnancy outcomes and reduce side effects, it has been received with mixed results (18-32). It also requires simultaneous coordination of two professionals, the physician who performs the transfer and the ultrasonographer (29). Furthermore, all transcervical and transmyometrial techniques involve "blind" introduction of the embryo(s) via transfer catheters with no real time flexibility of the tip of the transfer catheter and subsequent release of embryo(s) onto the surface of the endometrium. As a result if the embryo fails to adhere, due to some luteal phase defect or other, undefined "implantation window" problem, there is a significant risk that the embryo might be washed out of the cervix or become lodged in the fallopian tubes. In part, to compensate for this potential conceptus loss, physicians have adopted the practice of transferring higher numbers of embryos back to the uterus. Here we re-investigate the potential of surgical implantation of embryos developed to the blastocyst stage *in vitro* by day 5 or 6 post insemination. It does appear that this procedure may enable circumvention of those problems associated with the maternal receptivity aspect of the so called "window of implantation"(4). Under normal, non-assisted, circumstances, implantation begins six to seven days post ovulation. It involves multiple steps which can be summarized as pre-attachment, attachment-invasion, and decidualization - early placentation (33, 34). The reader is referred to a recent paper by Dominguez et al. (2) for a comprehensive review. Thus far, mechanisms for repairing defects in this process or clinically relevant markers of uterine receptivity have proven elusive. Similarly to the now well-accepted procedure of ICSI (35), where a single sperm is mechanically injected into an oocyte, with the development of this project we aim to develop an instrument and procedure whereby "mechanical" implantation of the embryo is achieved.

Ectopic Pregnancies after IVF specially for tubal disease account for approximately 8-10% of pregnancies (7, 48). Hysteroscopic SEED minimizes the chances of "losing" the embryo, and virtually eliminates ectopic pregnancies (tubal, placenta previa, cervical, or heterotopic) from embryo transfer, as the embryo(s) is embedded into the endometrium and not floating in the uterus. Using the flexible mini-hysteroscope affords an objective and accurate confirmation of the placement of the embryo that should make the procedure replicable, and thus more reliable with more consistent and improved results. Allowing the embryos to reach the blastocyst stage prior to transfer is gaining more acceptance (37-39). It allows both for more normal embryos to be naturally selected and for a more accurate selection of more viable, healthier embryo(s) (40-42). Thus a less number of embryos can be selected for transfer with more certainty for a successful singleton pregnancy (43, 44). This is congruent with the results in this study where there were no multiple pregnancies from day 6 implantations (Table 1).

A previous report on the use of SEED technique documented a promising set of results in patients with a variety of reasons for IVF (36). In this report we wanted to focus on a specific group of patients to better define the role of SEED technique. An overall pregnancy rate of 67% with a live birth rate of 29% was achieved. This is consistent with treating a better prognostic group of patients, i.e. egg donors in contrast with a non selective group of patients (36).

A possible drawback with the transcervical hysteroscopic embryo implantation (SEED) is the potential to scratch the endometrium and trigger some deleterious effect. Yet this is a potential hazard of "blind" procedures as well. The risk of disruption of the uterine lining, however is postulated to be less than "blind" and ultrasound guided transfers due to the advantage of direct visualization of the uterine lining and not requiring movement of the catheter to facilitate identification during ultrasound (32). As opposed to rigid endoscopes which may cause trauma to the uterus, the hysteroscope used in this study is a mini-hysteroscope with a 3mm diameter and flexible tip that allows one to easily follow the curvature of the uterus. With this protocol, though, the physician may then choose a non-scratched portion of the endometrium for implantation. Having said that, a growing number of literature suggests that mild inflammation may very well facilitate, if not be required for implantation and placentation (45-47).

Likewise, visualizing implantation allows for the physician to avoid losing embryos due to intrinsic uterine contractions or those brought on by the transfer, enabling the physician to defer the procedure until the enhanced activity has subsided. Furthermore, visualization allows one to place the embryo at a different location if trauma ensues. Also, the catheter used is semi-rigid to prevent kinking as it passes through the endoscope yet with enough flexibility to bend with the endoscope however bend and become kinked to prevent inadvertent passage into the myometrium. In addition, the uterine cavity is allowed to be distended during introduction of the hysteroscope into the uterus by slow passage through the endocervical canal. This would allow the hysteroscope to move in a gaseous space and not in direct contact with the endometrium as is the case with the blind procedure. In our study, no disruption to the uterine lining or uterine bleeding occurred. Increased cost is another drawback, however utilizing a hysteroscope with an objective replicable procedure that improves results will decrease the costs from multiple failed IVF-ET attempts and improve patient satisfaction.

5. Conclusion

We suggest that using a hysteroscopic subendometrial embryo delivery (SEED) for transferring advanced blastocyst(s) is a reasonable and effective method of embryo transfer. It will virtually eliminate ectopic pregnancies of all locations, i.e. tubal pregnancies as well as placenta previa, cervical, and heterotopic pregnancies, from IVF. Furthermore, it would allow for a targeted objective, reliable, safe and replicable method for single embryo transfer, as new and improved techniques along with modified media for handling, culture, and selection of embryos are introduced. This would greatly alleviate the anxiety, and cost to the patient as it decreases the number of attempts at using IVF in achieving a successful singleton pregnancy.

Author details

Michael Kamrava and Mei Yin
West Coast IVF Clinic, Inc., Beverly Hills, California, USA

Acknowledgement

Supported by West Coast IVF Clinic, Inc. and LA IVF Lab, LLC, Beverly Hills, CA USA

6. References

[1] Sharkey AM, Smith SK. The endometrium as a cause of implantation failure. Best Pract Res Clin Obstet Gynaecol 2003;17:289-307.

[2] Dominguez F, Avila S, Cervero A, Martin J, Pellicer A, Castrillo JL, Simon C. A combined approach for gene discovery identifies insulin-like growth factor-binding

protein-related protein 1 as a new gene implicated in human endometrial receptivity. J Clin Endocrinol Metab 2003;88:1849-57.

[3] Jokimaa V, Oksjoki S, Kujari H, Vuorio E, Anttila L. Altered expression of genes involved in the production and degradation of endometrial extracellular matrix in patients with unexplained infertility and recurrent miscarriages. Mol Hum Reprod 2002;8:1111-6.

[4] Kabir-Salmani M, Murphy C, Hosseini A, Valojerdi M. Ultrastructural Modifications of Human Endometrium during the Window of Implantation. IJFS 2:2008:44-59

[5] Sharif K, Afnan M, Lenton W, Bilalis D, Hunjan M, Khalaf Y. Transmyometrial embryo transfer after difficult immediate mock transcervical transfer. Fertil Steril 1996;65:1071-4.

[6] Mansour RT, Aboulghar MA, Serour GI, Amin YM. Dummy embryo transfer using methylene blue dye. Hum Reprod 1994;9:1257-9.

[7] Velalopoulou A. Ectopic Pregnancy and assisted reproductive technologies: A systematic review. Ectopic Pregnancy, Modern management and diagnosis Intech 2011; 45-78.

[8] Biervliet FP, Lesny P, Maguiness SD, Robinson J, Killick SR. Transmyometrial embryo transfer and junctional zone contractions. Hum Reprod 2002;17:347-50.

[9] Ghazzawi IM, Al-Hasani S, Karaki R, Souso S. Transfer technique and catheter choice influence the incidence of transcervical embryo expulsion and the outcome of IVF. Hum Reprod 1999;14:677-82.

[10] Groutz A, Lessing JB, Wolf Y, Azem F, Yovel I, Amit A. Comparison of transmyometrial and transcervical embryo transfer in patients with previously failed in vitro fertilization-embryo transfer cycles and/or cervical stenosis. Fertil Steril 1997;67:1073-6.

[11] Nakayama T, Goto Y, Kanzaki H, Takabatake K, Himeno T, Noda Y, Mori T. The use of intra-endometrial embryo transfer for increasing the pregnancy rate. Hum Reprod 1995;10:1833-6.

[12] Asaad M, Carver-Ward JA. Twin pregnancy following transmyometrial-subendometrial embryo transfer for repeated implantation failure. Hum Reprod 1997;12:2824-5.

[13] Itskovitz-Eldor J, Filmar S, Manor D, Stein D, Lightman A, Kol S. Assisted implantation: direct intraendometrial embryo transfer. Gynecol Obstet Invest 1997;43:73-5.

[14] Wimalasundera RC, Trew G, Fisk NM. Reducing the incidence of twins and triplets. Best Pract Res Clin Obstet Gynaecol 2003;17:309-29.

[15] Pasqualini RS, Quintans CJ. Clinical practice of embryo transfer. Reprod Biomed Online 2002;4:83-92.

[16] Choe JK, Nazari A, Check JH, Summers-Chase D, Swenson K. Marked improvement in clinical pregnancy rates following in vitro fertilization-embryo transfer seen when transfer technique and catheter were changed. Clin Exp Obstet Gynecol 2001;28:223-224.

[17] Schoolcraft WB, Surrey ES, Gardner DK. Embryo transfer: techniques and variables affecting success. Fertil Steril 2001;76:863-870.

[18] Lambers MJ, Dogan E, Kostelijk H, Lens JW, Schats R, Hompes PGA. Ultrasonographic-guided embryo transfer does not enhance pregnancy rates compared with embryo transfer based on previous uterine length measurement. Fertil Steril. 2006; 86: 867-872.

[19] Flisser E, Grifo JA. Is what we clearly see really so obvious? Ultrasonography and transcervical embryo transfer - a review. Fertil Steril. 2007; 87: 1-5.

[20] Allahbadia G, Gandhi G, Athavale U, Merchant R, Virk SPS, Kaur K. A blind embryo transfer is a rate limiting step to successful IVF. Fertil Steril. 2002: 78 Suppl 1: S157-S158.

[21] Puerto B, Creus M, Carmona F, Cívico S, Vanrell JA, Balasch J. Ultrasonography as a predictor of embryo implantation after in vitro fertilization: a controlled study. Fertil Steril. 2003; 79: 1015-1022.

[22] Tiras B, Polat M, Korucuoglu U, Zeyneloglu HB, Yarali H. Impact of embryo replacement depth on in vitro fertilization and embryo transfer outcomes. Fertil Steril. 2009; 7: 1666.

[23] Flisser E, Grifo JA,. Krey LC, Noyes N. Transabdominal ultrasound - assisted embryo transfer and pregnancy outcome. Fertil Steril. 2006; 85: 353-357.

[24] Gergely RZ, Danzer H, Surrey M, Hill D. Maximal implantation potential (MIP) pointsuggested target for optimal embryo placement within the uterine cavity during embryo transfer. Fertil Steril. 2007; 88(1): S328.

[25] Allahbadia GN, Kadam K, Gandhi G, Arora S, Valliappan JB, Joshi A, et al. Embryo transfer using the SureView catheter-beacon in the womb. Fertil Steril. 2010; 93: 344-350.

[26] Anderson RE, Nugent NL, Gregg AT, Nunn SL, Behr BR. Transvaginal ultrasoundguided embryo transfer improves outcome in patients with previous failed in vitro fertilization cycles. Fertil Steril. 2002; 77: 769-775.

[27] Kol S. Ultrasound-guided embryo transfer - a special role in patients with certain uterine defects. Fertil Steril. 2008; 89: 260.

[28] Kiltz RJ, Woodhouse D, Restive L, Miller D, Sciera A, Fundalinski J. Vaginal vs. abdominal ultrasound guidance for embryo transfer. Fertil Steril. 2006; 86 Suppl 1: S245-S246.

[29] Gergely RZ, DeUgarte CM, Danzer H, Surrey M, Hill D, DeCherney AH. Three dimensional/four dimensional ultrasound-guided embryo transfer using the maximal implantation potential point. Fertil Steril. 2005; 84: 500- 503.

[30] Pinto AB, Wright JD, Keller SL, Odem RR, Ratts VS,. William DB. Ultrasound guided embryo transfer in selected patients undergoing IVF. Fertil Steril. 2002; 77(3): S19.

[31] Abou-Setta AM, Mansour RT, Al-Inany HG, Aboulghar MM, Aboulghar MA, Serour GI. Among women undergoing embryo transfer, is the probability of pregnancy and live birth improved with ultrasound guidance over clinical touch alone? A systemic review and metaanalysis of prospective randomized trials. Fertil Steril. 2007; 88: 333-341.

[32] Frattarelli JL, Miller KL. The pre-cycle blind mock transfer is an inaccurate predictor of anticipated embryo transfer depth. Fertil Steril. 2006; 86(3): S184.

[33] Morrish DW, Dakour J, Li H. Life and death in the placenta: new peptides and genes regulating human syncytiotrophoblast and extravillous cytotrophoblast lineage formation and renewal. Curr Protein Pept Sci. 2001; 2:245-59.
[34] Giudice LC. Genes associated with embryonic attachment and implantation and the role of progesterone. J Reprod Med. 1999; 44: 165-71.
[35] Payne D. Embryo viability associated with microassisted fertilization. Baillieres Clin Obstet Gynaecol.1994; 8: 157-75.
[36] Kamrava, M, Yin M. Hysteroscopic Subendometrial Embryo Delivery (SEED), Mechanical Embryo Implantation. International Journal of Fertility and Sterility. Vol 4, No 1, Apr-Jun 2010, Pages: 29-34
[37] Shapiro BS, Daneshmand ST, Garner FC, Aguirre M, Hudson C, Thomas S. High ongoing pregnancy rates after deferred transfer through bipronuclear oocyte cryopreservation and post-thaw extended culture. Fertil Steril. 2009; 92: 1594-1599.
[38] Goto S, Kadowaki T, Hashimoto H, Kokeguchi S, Shiotani M. Stimulation of endometrium embryo transfer can improve implantation and pregnancy rates for patients undergoing assisted reproductive technology for the first time with a high-grade blastocyst. Fertil Steril. 2009; 92: 1264-1268.
[39] Lin PY, Huang FJ, Kung FT, Wang LI, Chang SY, Lan KC. Comparison of the offspring sex ratio between fresh and vitrificationthawed blastocyst transfer. Fertil Steril. 2009; 92: 1764-1766.
[40] Okimura T, Kuwayama M, Segawa T, Takehara Y, Kato K, Kato O. Relations between the timing of transfer, expansion size and implantation rates in frozen thawed single blastocyst transfer. Fertil Steril. 2009; 92(3 Suppl 1): S246.
[41] Stevens J, Schoolcraft WB, Schlenker T, Wagley L, Munne S, Gardner DK. Day 3 Blastomere Biopsy Does Not Affect Subsequent Blastocyst Development or Implantation Rate. Fertil Steril. 2000; 74 Suppl 1: S173.
[42] Weston G, Osianlis T, Catt J, Vollenhoven B. Blastocyst transfer does not cause a sexratio imbalance. Fertil Steril. 92: 1302-1305.
[43] Stillman RJ, Richter KS, Banks NK, Graham JR. Elective single embryo transfer: A 6-year progressive implementation of 784 single blastocyst transfers and the influence of payment method on patient choice. Fertil Steril. 2009; 92: 1895-1906.
[44] Sparks AE, Ryan GL, Sipe CS, Dokras AJ, Syrop CH, Van Voorhis BJ. Reducing the risk of multi-fetal gestation by implementation of a single blastocyst transfer policy. Fertil Steril. 2005; 84(Suppl 1): S86-S87.
[45] Johnson GA, Burghardt RC, Bazer FW, Spencer TE. Osteopontin: roles in implantation and placentation. Biol Reprod. 2003; 69(5): 1458-1471.
[46] Barash A, Dekel N, Fieldust S, Segal I, Schechtman E, Granot I. Local injury to the endometrium doubles the incidence of successful pregnancies in patients undergoing in vitro fertilization. Fertil Steril. 2003; 79: 1317- 1322.
[47] Wilcox AJ, Weinberg CR, O'Connor JF, Baird DD, Schlatterer JP, Canfield RE, et al. Incidence of early loss of pregnancy. N Engl J Med. 1988; 319: 189-194.

[48] Ketefian A, Sproul K, Buyalos R, Hubert G, Kumar A. Ectopic Pregnancy (EP) after In Vitro Fertilization (IVF) and Subsequent Pregnancy Outcomes. Fert Steril. 2007 vol 87 suppl 2, S16-17.

Chapter 7

Luteal Phase Support in ART: An Update

Mohamad E. Ghanem and Laila A. Al-Boghdady

Additional information is available at the end of the chapter

http://dx.doi.org/10.5772/51093

1. Introduction

Assisted reproductive techniques (ART) as defined by ICMART (international society of monitoring assisted reproduction) and WHO is all treatments or procedures that include the in vitro handling of both human oocytes and sperm or of embryos for the purpose of establishing a pregnancy. This includes, but is not limited to, in vitro fertilization (IVF)/intracytoplasmic sperm injection (ICSI) and embryo transfer, gamete intrafallopian transfer, zygote intrafallopian transfer, tubal embryo transfer, gamete and embryo cryopreservation, oocytes and embryo donation, and gestational surrogacy. ART does not include assisted insemination (artificial insemination) using sperm from either a woman's partner or a sperm donor [1]. On the other hand the term medically assisted reproduction (MAR) is given to the wider scope involving reproductive ovarian stimulation with or without insemination and ART techniques mentioned above [1]

The luteal phase is defined as the period from occurrence of ovulation until the establishment of a pregnancy or the resumption of menses 2 weeks later. In the context of assisted reproduction techniques luteal phase support (LPS) is the term used to describe the administration of medications with the aim to support the process of implantation.

2. Pathophysiology of luteal phase in ART

Progesterone and estrogen are required to prepare the uterus for embryo implantation and to modulate the endometrium during the early stages of pregnancy. In the normal luteal phase of a nonpregnant woman, steroid production peaks four days after ovulation and continues for one week until falling several days before the next menses. If pregnancy occurs, progesterone production is restored by human chorionic gonadotrophin (hCG) stimulation. Once the oocyte is released, the follicle collapses and the remaining granulosa cells, which have acquired receptors for luteinizing hormone (LH), rapidly undergo luteinisation under the influence of LH. The formed corpus luteum requires regular stimulation by LH to maintain adequate production of progesterone [2].The absence of LH due to pituitary suppression by gonadotropin releasing hormone (GnRh) analogues deprives the corpus luteum from this LH.

In the mid-1980s, the incorporation of GnRh agonists into ovarian stimulation regimens became associated with improved outcomes after IVF and other assisted reproduction technologies. Pituitary function does not resume completely until 2–3 weeks after the end of GnRH-agonist therapy; and luteal phase support was considered essential to counter any luteal insufficiency that may have a negative impact on an early pregnancy [3 ,4]. It is well established that luteal function is compromised in IVF cycles [5, 6, 7]. The reasons for luteal phase abnormalities in ART are multiple. It has been shown that the function of the corpus luteum is compromised by the process of follicular aspiration for oocyte retrieval as granulosa cells are mechanically disrupted and aspirated. The severity of the disruption seems to be in relation to the vigorousness and the number of aspirations and therefore the number of granulosa cells that are dislodged from the membrana granulosa layer [8].It has been proved that luteal phase defect occurs in long GnRh-agonist protocol [9] and that corpus luteum deficiency as sequel of assisted reproduction techniques in general , is partially caused by aspiration of the granulosa cells and the use of gonadotropin-releasing hormone agonists. Due to the immediate recovery of pituitary gonadotrophin release just after discontinuation of the GnRH antagonists, it has been hypothesized that the luteal phase would be less disturbed in these cycles [10]. Although preliminary observations in intrauterine insemination cycles favored this contention, studies on a limited number of cases undergoing IVF demonstrated that there was a significant reduction in pregnancy rates without luteal phase support [11]. The serum LH levels in the early and midluteal phase of GnRH antagonist–treated cycles were low, regardless of the regimen used to induce oocyte maturation [12]. In the absence of luteal phase support, the area under the curve for progesterone was suboptimal and this was accompanied by premature luteolysis [13]. In nonsupported cycles, the length of the luteal phase was shortened and early bleeding occurred [14]. Based on this body of evidence, luteal phase support should be considered in IVF cycles where GnRH antagonists are used.

Other causes of the luteal phase defect observed in stimulated IVF cycles are related to the multifollicular development achieved during ovarian stimulation. This leads to supra-physiological concentrations of steroids secreted by a high number of corpora lutea during the early luteal phase, which directly inhibit LH release via negative feedback actions at the hypothalamic - pituitary axis level, rather than a central pituitary cause or steroidogenic abnormality in the corpus luteum [15].As previously alluded to, luteal phase defect in IVF is present whether GnRH agonist or antagonist is used [16]. Many meta-analyses concurred that luteal support improves IVF outcome [17, 18 ,19 ,20, 21].The most recent Cochraine review [21] confirmed earlier studies and found that luteal phase support with hCG provided significant benefit as compared to placebo or no treatment, with a significant increase in ongoing pregnancy rate and a decrease in miscarriage rate when GnRH agonist was used. Luteal phase support with progesterone, compared to placebo or no treatment in GnRH agonist and non-GnRH agonist cycles, also resulted in a significant increase in clinical pregnancy rates and live birth.

3. Options of luteal support in ART

To correct the luteal phase defect in stimulated IVF/ICSI cycles, progesterone and /or human chorionic gonadotrophin (hCG) can be administered. The addition of estardiol to progesterone luteal support is currently debated and the final situation in luteal phase support needs further studies. The use of GnRh agonist in luteal support has been recommended in more recent studies.

4. Progesterone

Progesterone produced by the corpus luteum causes the secretory transformation of the endometrium that is necessary for implantation and for the early development of the fertilized ovum. In response to progesterone, the glands become tortuous and secretory and there is an increase in stromal vascularity, thus making the endometrium both morphologically and functionally well prepared for implantation. Progesterone preparations can be divided into two groups: natural progesterone and synthetic preparations. Synthetic derivatives or progestins are 1) 17-hydroxyprogesterone derivatives and 2) 19-nortestosterone derivatives. The 19-nortestosterone synthetic derivatives resist enzymatic degradation if given orally, but have a high incidence of secondary effects and have been associated with mood changes, depression, virilization, decreases in high-density lipoproteins, luteolysis and a possibly teratogenic effect that limits their use during fertile cycles. Natural progesterone has no adverse effects on high-density lipoproteins, no teratogenic effects and is more effective than the derivatives in inducing secretory changes at the endometrium (22). Traditionally, progesterone was given by means of intramuscular injections, what makes it unacceptable for long-term treatment. In this respect the vaginal route is the preferred way to administer natural progesterone.

Various formulations of progesterone are now available, including oral, vaginal, and intramuscular (I.M) progesterone . Parenteral administration of progesterone, vaginally or I.M, does not subject the compound to the significant metabolic consequences of oral administration. Progesterone administered orally is subjected to first-pass pre-hepatic and hepatic metabolism. This metabolic activity results in progesterone degradation to its 5α- and 5β-reduced metabolites [23] . Levine and Watson [24] compared the pharmacokinetics of an oral micronized progesterone preparation (Prome- trium, 100 mg, Solvay Pharmaceuticals Inc., Marietta, GA) with that of a vaginal progesterone gel (Crinone 8%, 90 mg).Results showed that the vaginal gel was associated with a higher maximum serum concentration of progesterone. Furthermore, the 24-hour area under the curve for drug concentration vs. time (AUC0–24) was higher in the group that had received the vaginal preparation. This signifies greater total progesterone exposure over 24 hours for a single dose of progesterone administered in a vaginal gel compared with a similar dose administered orally. Levine and Watson [24] concluded that the vaginal administration of progesterone results in a greater bioavailability with less relative variability than oral progesterone. There are no agreement on the standard dose of progesterone in luteal phase support. Studies have been conducted using I.M. injections

(12.5–100 mg/day), various vaginal preparations such as creams, pessaries, sustained release gel and vaginal rings, vaginal applications of oral formulations and oral preparations including micronized progesterone (600–1200 mg/day) and dydrogesterone (oral, 20–30 mg/day) [25].

4.1. Comparison between routes of progesterone administration

Progesterone can be administered orally, vaginally, or through I.M. injection and all these routes of administration have demonstrated characteristic endometrial histological changes [26]. Oral dosing requires a higher concentration in order to compensate for "first-pass" liver metabolism. The bioavailability of the orally administered progesterone can be as low as 10% [27].Micronized dosage forms of progesterone are utilized to increase efficiency of delivery. Micronization decreases particle size and shortens its dissolution time according to the equation of Noyes - Whitney[28].However, oral administration may result in noticeable sedative and anxiolytic effects due to progesterone metabolites that enhance inhibitory neurotransmission by binding to the $GABA_A$ receptor complex [29].

Intramuscular injections of micronized progesterone in oil result in a higher peak and longer lasting plasma concentrations when compared to aqueous solutions. But, a daily administration is required due to a rapid metabolism. Progesterone in oil (USP) is formulated with sesame oil (50 mg/ml) and 10% v/v benzyl alcohol that functions as preservative. Intramuscular injections are difficult to self-administer and are often painful. A common practice is to warm up the oil solution in order to decrease its viscosity in an attempt to reduce pain with injection [28].

Bulletti et al[30] first described a preferential trafficking of vaginally delivered progesterone to the uterus leading to a higher progesterone concentration in the endometrial tissue compared to the blood serum. Therefore, targeted delivery of progesterone directly to the uterus is thus achievable through utilizing this 'uterine first pass effect' [31] .The anatomy of the vagina with its rich vascular plexus provides an ideal environment for absorbing drugs. The rugae of the vaginal wall increase the total available surface area. The vascular system around the vagina and the venous drainage of the vagina does not initially pass through the liver, and thus bypasses the first pass hepatic effect [32] .By avoiding the hepatic first pass effect, vaginal progesterone does not create high concentrations of metabolites that cause undesired side effects. Vaginal administration of progesterone results in more consistent serum levels, which can remain elevated for up to 48

4.2. Oral dydrogesterone vs. vaginal micronized progesterone

In a prospective randomized study [33] a total of 430 women underwent IVF/ICSI treatment. Long protocol gonadotropin releasing hormone analogue down-regulation was followed by gonadotropin stimulation. Luteal support was initiated from the day of embryo transfer and continued for up to 14 days. Patients were randomised to luteal supplementation with either intravaginal micronised progesterone 200 mg three times daily (n = 351) or oral dydrogesterone 10mg twice daily (n = 79). In cases of a positive pregnancy test, luteal support was continued for 12 weeks. Both dydrogesterone and micronised progesterone were associated with similar rates of successful pregnancies. Vaginal discharge or irritation were reported by 10.5% of patients given micronized progesterone. Significantly ($p < 0.05$), more patients given dydrogesterone than micronised progesterone were satisfied with the tolerability of their treatment. There were no differences between the treatments with regard to liver function tests. In agreement with this another study [34] compared oral dydrogesterone for luteal-phase support in assisted reproductive technologies with micronized vaginal progesterone. All patients underwent long-term downregulation with gonadotropin-releasing hormone agonists. In phase I, 498 patients were divided into three groups: long protocol and not at risk of OHSS (group A); long protocol and at risk of OHSS (group B); and those in a donor oocyte program (group C). All patients received micronized progesterone 600 mg/day, vaginally. They were also randomized to dydrogesterone 20 mg/day (n = 218) or placebo (n = 280). The pregnancy rate was higher with dydrogesterone than with placebo in group A (33.0% vs. 23.6%), group B (36.8% vs. 28.1%) and group C (42.9% vs. 15.6%; $p < 0.001$). In phase II, 675 patients were divided into the same three groups (groups D, E and F) and were randomized to dydrogesterone 30 mg/day (n = 366) or micronized progesterone 600 mg/day (n = 309). The pregnancy rate was significantly higher with dydrogesterone than with progesterone in group D (39.1% vs. 26.7%; $p < 0.01$), group E (41.2% vs. 35.6%; $p < 0.01$) and group F (48.2% vs. 33.9%; $p < 0.001$).Although both routes had more or less comparable cycle outcome the cited studies did not comment on sedative effects of oral synthetic dydrogesterone compared with vaginal micronized progesterone.

4.3. Micronized progesterone: oral vs. vaginal routes

A prospective randomized small sample study [35] compared the efficacy of micronized progesterone administered as luteal support following ovulation induction for in-vitro fertilization (IVF)– embryo transfer in cycles using gonadotrophin-releasing hormone agonist, orally (200 mg×4/day) or vaginally (100 mg×2/day) and to characterize the luteal phase hormonal profile during such treatments. A total of 64 high responder patients requiring intracytoplasmic sperm injection due to male factor infertility were prospectively randomized into two treatment groups. Patients treated orally or vaginally were comparable in age, number of oocytes retrieved, and number of embryos transferred per cycle. Following low dose vaginal treatment, a significantly higher implantation rate (30.7 versus 10.7%, $P < 0.01$), and a tendency to higher clinical pregnancy rate (47.0 versus 33.3%) and ongoing pregnancy rate (41.1 versus 20.0%) was observed, compared with oral treatment. In conception cycles, luteal serum progesterone and oestrogen concentrations did not differ between the treatment groups. In non-conception cycles, late luteal progesterone concentrations were significantly lower following vaginal treatment. As low dose micronized progesterone administered vaginally is simple, easy and well tolerated, it could be recommended as the method of choice for luteal support.

4.4. Oral micronized progesterone vs. I.M progesterone

Oral micronized progesterone for luteal phase support in ART not only results in significantly lower rates of pregnancy and implantation compared with those for I.M. , hCG or progesterone, but also causes more side effects [36] .In a prospective randomized study, the implantation rate was significantly lower in the oral micronized progesterone arm compared with I.M. progesterone. There was no significant difference in pregnancy rate between both groups [37] As mentioned above parenteral administration of progesterone, vaginally or I.M, does not subject the compound to the significant metabolic consequences of oral administration. Progesterone administered orally is subjected to first-pass pre-hepatic and hepatic metabolism [23].

4.5. Vaginal vs. IM progesterone for luteal support

Previous randomized trials [38 ,39] and a meta-analysis [18] and a Cochrane review [19] concluded that there is evidence of superiority of I.M. over vaginal progesterone for ongoing pregnancy and live birth. These studies showed that whether natural or synthetic I.M progesterone were used the results were the same : superiority of I.M. over vaginal ` progesterone For example at least two prospective randomized trials [40,41] showed that biweekly I.M. 250 mg 17-alpha hydroxyl progesterone caproate (17 –αHPC) was superior to daily 90 mg vaginal gel. However more recent randomized trials [42 ,43] and Cochrane systematic reviews found no evidence favoring vaginal vs. I.M. administration of progesterone. The last Cochrain review and meta-analysis [21] is particularly relevant because it is the most recent (2011) and it included Sixty-nine studies with a total of 16,327 women.

5. Comparison of different vaginal progesterone preparations

Natural progesterone have been incorporated in different forms for vaginal adminstration.e.g. vaginal tablets or capsules , vaginal pessaries and vaginal gel. The tablets adsorb the vaginal secretions and disintegrate into an adhesive powder that adheres to the vaginal epithelium, thus facilitating sustained absorption and reduced perineal irritation [44]. Each vaginal insert delivers 100 mg of progesterone in a base containing excipients conventionally used for solid oral dosage forms: lactose monohydrate, polyvinylpyrrolidone, adipic acid, sodium bicarbonate, sodium lauryl sulfate, magnesium stearate, pregelatinized starch, and colloidal silicone dioxide. Vaginal suppositories (e.g. Cyclogest)., contain semi-synthetic glycerides produced from interesterification of hydrogenated vegetable oil. The carrier vehicle in gel preparations (e.g. Crinone) is an oil-in-water emulsion containing polycarbophil, a bioadhesive and water-swellable polymer [28]. The water phase bypasses dependence on the local vaginal moisture, which is highly variable. The progesterone is sparingly soluble in oil (1:30 w/w) and practically insoluble in water (1:10,000 w/w) therefore the majority of the progesterone exists in a suspended form. The emulsion containing both dissolved and suspended progesterone adheres to the vaginal epithelial cells and thereafter-dissolved progesterone permeates through the mucosal tissue. The depletion of dissolved progesterone in the formulation is replenished by the dissolution of suspended progesterone particles

5.1. Pessaries vs. capsules

A prospective randomized study [45] compared the luteal serum hormone level, effectiveness and tolerability of two different vaginal formulations of micronized progesterone, vaginal pessaries (Ellios) and capsules (Uterogestan) , used for luteal phase support after an in vitro fertilization (IVF). Patients received Ellios pessaries (2 times 200-mg pessary/day) or Utrogestan capsules (2 100-mg capsules, two times a day). Progesterone was administered from the day of oocyte pickup (day 0) until menses or up to 10 weeks in pregnant patients. The outcome measures showed that progesterone levels on days 0, 9, 16 were not statistically different between the two formulations. The pregnancy rate were similar in the two groups (25.5% vs. 18.6%), whereas tolerance was significantly better in pessaries` group versus capsules` group (vaginal discharge: 43% vs. 82%).

5.2. Suppositories vs. tablets

Another randomized trial [46] compared side effects and patient convenience of vaginal progesterone suppositories (Cyclogest) and vaginal progesterone tablets (Endometrin) used for luteal phase support in in vitro fertilization/embryo transfer cycles using pituitary. downregulation. One hundred and thirty-two infertile patients were randomized on the day of embryo transfer by a computer-generated randomization list in sealed envelopes to receive either Cyclogest 400 mg or Endometrin 100 mg twice daily for 14 days. On days 6 and 16 after ET, they rated side effects and patient convenience into four grades: none, mild, moderate and severe by completing a questionnaire.The results showed no significant differences in perineal irritation on days 6 and 16 after embryo transfer between the two groups, although there was a trend of fewer patients with perineal irritation in the Endometrin group. Significantly more patients in the Endometrin group had difficulty of administration on day 6 after embryo transfer. There were no differences in the hormonal profile on day 6 after embryo transfer and IVF outcomes between the two groups. The study concluded that there was no difference in perineal irritation after the use of Cyclogest suppositories or Endometrin tablets for luteal phase support although more patients found administration of Endometrin tablets difficult.

5.3. Gel vs. capsule

The first prospective randomized trial comparing vaginal cream Crinone 8% [47] investigated 126 patients undergoing cycles of IVF / ICSI. Patients received either Crinone 8% (n = 73) vaginally once daily or two Utrogest capsules (n=53) vaginally three times daily (600 mg). Clinical pregnancy rates were comparable (28.8 versus 18.9%), as were clinical abortion rates until 12 weeks of gestation (14.3 versus 10.0%) and clinical ongoing pregnancy rates (24.7 versus 17.0%) in the Crinone 8% and Utrogest groups, respectively.

Forty-seven non-pregnant patients were randomly selected to answer questions regarding comfort during luteal phase support. Crinone 8% had a clear advantage over Utrogest as it resulted in less vaginal discharge ($P < 0.01$) and fewer application difficulties ($P<0.05$). Twenty patients familiar with the alternative preparation from a previous cycle also noted that Crinone 8% was easier to apply ($P < 0.01$) and less time consuming ($P < 0.05$) to use than Utrogest. In another prospective multicenter randomized trial [48] to study the comparative efficacy and tolerability of capsules containing 200 mg of progesterone (Utrogest 200) or Crinone 8% gel for luteal phase and early pregnancy support during assisted reproduction techniques.Four hundred thirty women who underwent their first IVF or ICSI cycle were randomized after successful transfer of two or three embryos. Patients used vaginally applied capsules containing 200 mg of progesterone (Utrogest 200) three times per day or containing Crinone 8% gel twice per day. Therapy was started in the evening of the embryo transfer day and continued up to 10 weeks in pregnant women. If the pregnancy test proved to be negative, application was stopped. The luteal phase support in ART cycles with Utrogest™ 200 capsules (three times per day) or Crinone 8% gel (two times per day) by the vaginal route resulted in similar outcomes with respect to implantation, ongoing pregnancy, and abortion rates. The two recommended regimens of progesterone supplementation in ART proved to be equivalent and safe. A large prospective randomized study [49] compared the efficacy of intravaginal and I.M. progesterone for luteal phase support in IVF cycles. The study included women 25-44 years old with infertility necessitating treatment with IVF, 511 consecutive patients were enrolled; 474 completed participation, and 37 were excluded. Patient received luteal phase support using either Crinone 8% or natural progesterone in oil starting 2 days following oocyte retrieval. The outcome measure was pregnancy and delivery rates stratified by patient age. The study showed that overall, patients who received vaginal progesterone had higher pregnancy (70.9% vs. 64.2%) and delivery (51.7% vs. 45.4%) rates than did patients who received IM progesterone. Patients <35 who received vaginal progesterone had significantly higher delivery rates (65.7% vs. 51.1%) than did patients who received IMP. There were no differences, regardless of age, in the rates of biochemical pregnancy, miscarriage, or ectopics. The study concluded that in younger patients undergoing IVF, support of the luteal phase with Crinone produces significantly higher pregnancy rates than does IMP. Crinone and I.M. progesterone appear to be equally efficacious in the older patient. In a meta-analysis of published studies comparing vaginal progesterone gel for luteal support [50] seven randomized controlled trials, involving 2,447 patients, were included in the analysis. Studies were included where vaginal progesterone gel 90 mg once or twice daily versus any other vaginal progesterone form for luteal phase support. The endpoint was clinical pregnancy rate. No difference was observed in the overall clinical pregnancy rate when comparing vaginal progesterone gel with any other vaginal progesterone form. Moreover, clinical pregnancy rates were similar in protocols using only GnRH agonists and when comparing vaginal gel with the traditional treatment of 200 mg×3 vaginal progesterone capsules. The study concluded that no significant difference exists between vaginal gel and all other vaginal progesterone forms in terms of clinical pregnancy rates.

6. GnRh –agonist Luteal support

The first report on the place of GnRh-agonist in luteal support [51] randomized patients undergoing IVF using GnRH antagonist protocol in which triggering ovulation was done by 10 000 IU of hCG and luteal phase support was done by 600 mg of vaginal micronized progesterone as compared with triggering ovulation by 200 μg nasal GnRHa followed by different doses of intranasal GnRH-a. They found that 100 μg of buserlin intranasal three times daily is equivalent to 600 mg vaginal progesterone concerning clinical pregnancy rate. In another study [52] six hundred women about to undergo ovarian stimulation for ICSI (300 using a long GnRH agonist protocol and 300 using a GnRH antagonist protocol) were enrolled in this study. Patients treated with each of these two protocols were randomly assigned to receive a single injection of GnRH agonist or placebo 6 days after ICSI. Implantation and live birth rates were the primary outcomes.The results of the study showed that administration of 0.1 mg of GnRH agonist triptorelin on day 6 after ICSI led to a significant improvement of implantation and live birth rates after ICSI as compared with placebo. In GnRH antagonist-treated ovarian stimulation cycles, luteal-phase GnRH agonist also increased ongoing pregnancy rate. Moreover, luteal-phase GnRH agonist administration increased luteal-phase serum hCG, estradiol and progesterone concentrations in both ovarian stimulation regimens. The study concluded that luteal-phase GnRH agonist administration enhances ICSI clinical outcomes after GnRH agonist- and GnRH antagonist-treated ovarian stimulation cycles, possibly by a combination of effects on the embryo and the corpus luteum. However in a more recent study [53] five hundred and seventy women undergoing embryo transfer following controlled ovarian stimulation with a long GnRH agonist protocol were included. In addition to routine luteal phase support with progesterone, women were randomized to receive a single 0.1 mg dose of triptorelin or placebo 6 days after ICSI. Randomization was done on the day of embryo transfer according to a computer generated randomization table. Ongoing pregnancy rate beyond 20th week of gestation was the primary outcome measure. The trial was powered to detect a 12% absolute increase from an assumed 38% ongoing pregnancy rate in the placebo group, with an alpha error level of 0.05 and a beta error level of 0.2. The results showed that there were 89 (31.2%) ongoing pregnancies in the GnRH agonist group, and 84 (29.5%) in the control group (absolute difference +1.7%, 95% confidence interval −5.8% to +9.2%). Implantation, clinical pregnancy and multiple pregnancy rates were likewise similar in the GnRH agonist and placebo groups. The study concluded that single 0.1 mg triptorelin administration 6 days after ICSI following ovarian stimulation with the long GnRH agonist protocol does not seem to result in an increase ≥12% in ongoing pregnancy rates. Despite this, several independent studies reported beneficial effects of GnRh-a as luteal support. [41,42,54, 55 ,56] . In the most recent Cochrane review [15] six studies (1646 women) investigated progesterone versus progesterone + GnRH-a. The authors subgrouped the studies for single-dose GnRH agonist and multiple-dose GnRh agonist. For the live birth, clinical pregnancy and ongoing pregnancy rate the results suggested a significant effect in favor of progesterone and GnRH-a. The Peto OR for the live birth rate was 2.44 (95% CI 1.62 to 3.67), for the clinical pregnancy rate was 1.36 (95% CI 1.11 to 1.66) and for the ongoing pregnancy rate was 1.31 (95% CI 1.03

to 1.67). The results for miscarriage and multiple pregnancy did not indicate a difference of effect. The authors concluded that there were significant results showing a benefit from addition of GnRH- a to progesterone for the outcomes of live birth, clinical pregnancy and ongoing pregnancy. In another recent systematic review and meta-analysis [57] six relevant RCTs were identified including a total of 2012 patients. The probability of live birth rate (risk difference : +16%, 95% CI: +10 to +22%) was significantly higher in patients who received GnRH agonist support compared with those who did not. The subgroup analysis according to the type of GnRH analogue used for LH suppression did not change the effect observed (studies in which GnRH agonist was used during ovarian stimulation, risk difference : +15%, 95% CI: +5 to +23%); (studies in which GnRH antagonist was used during ovarian stimulation, risk difference : +19%, 95% CI: +11 to +27%). The conclusion of the study was that the best available evidence suggests that GnRH agonist addition during the luteal phase significantly increases the probability of live birth rates.

7. Human chorionic gonadotropins (hCG)

The use of hCG is driven by the hypothesis that, in addition to progesterone and estrogen, the corpus luteum produces other hormones which are required for endometrial transformation and optimization of the conditions for embryo implantation and development. Some randomized trials supported the use of hCG for luteal support [58 ,59].However one randomized controlled trial [60] where patients at ovum pick –up were randomized to receive luteal support as either progesterone only or hCG only or combination of progesterone and hCG showed that there were no statistically significant differences with regard to the main outcome parameter, the clinical ongoing pregnancy rate .However using a standardized discomfort scale, there were more complaints towards the end of the luteal phase in the groups receiving hCG only or an additional injection of hCG, when compared to the progesterone only groups .The conclusion of the study was that progesterone only for luteal phase support leads to the same clinical ongoing pregnancy rate as hCG, but has no impact on the comfort of the patient. Furthermore two meta-analyses [18 ,19] found no statistically significant differences in clinical pregnancy, ongoing pregnancy, and miscarriage rates between progesterone and hCG. The odds ratio of OHSS was more than threefold higher when hCG was added to the luteal phase support regimen, confirming that progesterone alone is a better strategy. In the most recent Cochrane review and meta-analysis [21], 15 studies, including 2117 women investigated progesterone versus hCG regimens. The hCG regimens were sub grouped into comparisons of progesterone versus hCG and progesterone versus progesterone + hCG. The results did not indicate a difference of effect between the interventions, except for OHSS. Furthermore subgroup analysis of progesterone versus progesterone + hCG showed a significant benefit from progesterone (Peto OR 0.45, 95% CI 0.26 to 0.79).

8. Estrogen

The use of a GnRH agonist is an integral part of long protocols used in IVF/ICSI cycles and it results in pituitary suppression and luteal phase deficiency with decline in serum

E2 and progesterone 8 days after hCG administration for oocyte maturation. Earlier reports indicated that serum E2 concentrations severely drop at the end of the luteal phase [61]; therefore,a concern has been raised about an additional supply of E2 during luteal phase of IVF cycles. The role of E2 luteal support is still debated after more than a decade of use. Previous meta analysis [18] and an update [62] and more recent randomized trials [63, 64] reported beneficial effects of adding E2 to luteal progesterone support. In our study [63] two hundred seventy-four women undergoing first ICSI cycles were randomized after ovum pickup into three groups of luteal support . Group I received IM progesterone only, group II received progesterone plus oral E2 valerate, group III received progesterone plus hCG. Outcome measures were pregnancy rate, implantation rate, rates of multiple pregnancy and miscarriage, and midluteal serum E2 and progesterone, and midluteal E2: progesterone ratio. The results showed that the pregnancy and implantation rates were significantly higher in group II (E2 plus progesterone) compared to group I (I.M. progesterone only) and the miscarriage rate was significantly lower in group II compared with group I. Midluteal E2 was significantly higher in group II compared with group I. The decline in E2 after ovum pickup was lowest in group II, highest in group I.

On the other hand two meta- analyses [65, 66] has shown that the addition of E2 to progesterone for luteal phase support in IVF/ICSI cycles has no beneficial effects on pregnancy rates. The last meta- analyses commented that the data in the literature are limited and heterogeneous, precluding the extraction of clear and definite conclusions. Therefore further studies are needed to clarify the exact role of E2 luteal support in long agonist vs. antagonist , normal responder vs. high responder and low responders.

9. Timing of starting luteal support

In stimulated IVF/ICSI cycles, the steroid production in the first week after oocyte retrieval is likely to be well timed and more than sufficient, so the start of exogenous support is not apt to be critical within this window. It was reported that pregnancy rates were higher in IVF when progesterone was started three rather than six days after oocyte collection [67] .A randomized controlled trial [68] allocated 130 patients to start luteal support at hCG day and , 128 at egg retrieval day and 127 at day of embryo transfer. Ongoing pregnancy rate of 20.8% was found in the hCG-day group versus 22.7 and 23.6% in the other two groups, respectively. This study showed that , there is no difference between the three different times of start of luteal support.

10. Duration of luteal support

Theoretically, progesterone would be of benefit to only 'fill in the gap' between clearance of exogenously administered hCG and the increase in endogenous hCG production. As soon as endogenous hCG production increases, the corpus luteum secretes an appropriate amount of progesterone [69].However most IVF centers extend luteal support for varying durations after positive pregnancy test. A questionnaire concerning details of luteal phase support was returned from 21 leading centers worldwide [70]. Micronized vaginal progesterone was used in 16 centers, one center used oral micronized progesterone, three centers used 50 mg I.M. progesterone and one center used hCG. All centers started luteal phase support on day of oocyte retrieval or day of embryo transfer. Luteal phase support was stopped on the day of [beta] hCG (BhCG) in eight centers, 2 weeks after positive B hCG in four centers, 2–4 weeks after positive B hCG in five centers, at 9, 10 and 11 weeks of pregnancy in three centers and at 12 weeks in one center. Schmidt et al. [69] compared two groups of patients who used luteal phase support for 2 or 5 weeks. The ongoing pregnancy rate and the delivery rates were not significantly different. The same Danish group [71] conducted a prospective randomized study on 303 women who achieved pregnancy after IVF or ICSI. All were treated with the long protocol using GnRH agonist and given luteal support with 200 mg vaginal progesterone three times daily during 14 days from the day of transfer until the day of a positive hCG test. The study group (n = 150) withdrew vaginal progesterone from the day of positive hCG. The control group (n = 153) continued administration of vaginal progesterone during the next 3 weeks of pregnancy. The study showed that the number of miscarriages prior to and after week 7 of gestation was seven (4.6%) and 15 (10.0%) in the study group and five (3.3%) and 13 (8.5%) in the control group, respectively. The number of deliveries was 118 (78.7%) in the study group and 126 (82.4%) in the control group. The differences were not significant. This is the first randomized study to conclude that prolongation of progesterone supplementation in early pregnancy has no influence on the miscarriage rate, and thus no effect on the delivery rate and progesterone supplementation can safely be withdrawn at the time of a positive hCG test

11. Chapter summary

In contemporary ART, luteal phase progesterone supplementation is common practice. Various routes of administration have been developed, but most have proved to have limitations and some side effects. The use of oral progesterone is clearly inferior to intramuscular or vaginal administration and is associated with an increased rate of side effects due to its metabolites. While intramuscular delivery of progesterone continues to remain an option, an increasing number of fertility specialists prefer the vaginal route of delivery. At present, there are insufficient data for a direct comparison between intramuscular and vaginal progesterone therapy; therefore, physicians should be guided by their own clinical experience. Progesterone by whatever route or form can be started on ovum pickup day or within 48 hours, without significant differences in cycle outcome.

Luteal phase support with hCG is not superior to luteal phase support with progesterone. Supplementary administration of hCG brings no advantage when progesterone is administered . Luteal phase support with hCG increases the risk of OHSS as compared with progesterone. As yet, the role of estrogen supplementation therapy during the luteal phase of IVF cycles lacks enough evidence to be employed in routine practice. Combined luteal support using progesterone and GnRh-a showed benefit from addition of GnRH- a to progesterone for the outcomes of live birth, clinical pregnancy and ongoing pregnancy.

Author details

Mohamad E. Ghanem* and Laila A. Al-Boghdady
Mansoura Faculty of Medicine and Mansoura Integrated Fertility Center, Mansoura, Egypt

12. References

[1] Zegers-Hochschild, F. Adamson, G. D. de Mouzon, J. Ishihara, O. Mansour, R. Nygren, K. Sullivan E and. Vanderpoel, S for ICMART and WHO International Committee for Monitoring Assisted Reproductive Technology (ICMART) and the World Health Organization (WHO) revised glossary of ART terminology, Fertil Steril,2009;92:1520–4.

[2] Vande Wiele RL, Bogumil J, Dyrenfurth I, Mechanisms regulating the menstrual cycle in women. Recent Prog Horm Res 1970; 26:63–103.

[3] J Smitz, P Erard, M Camus et al. Pituitary gonadotrophin secretory capacity during the luteal phase in superovulation using GnRH-agonists and HMG in a desensitization or flare-up protocol Hum Reprod, 1992; 7:1225–1229

[4] J Smitz, C Bourgain, L Van Waesberghe, M Camus, P Devroey, A.C Van Steirteghem ,A prospective randomized study on estradiol valerate supplementation in addition to intravaginal micronized progesterone in buserelin and HMG-induced superovulation Hum Reprod, 1993; 8: 40–45

[5] Tavaniotou A, Smitz J, Bourgain C, Devroey P. Ovulation induction disrupts luteal phase function. Ann NY Acad Sci 2001; 943:55–63

[6] Fauser BC, Devroey P. Reproductive biology and IVF: ovarian stimulation and luteal phase consequences. Trends Endocrinol Metab 2003; 14:236–242

[7] Devroey P, Bourgain C, Macklon N, Fauser BC. Reproductive biology and IVF: ovarian stimulation and endometrial receptivity. Trends Endocrinol Metab 2004; 15:84–90

[8] Garcia J, Jones GS, Acosta AA, Wright GL Jr. Corpus luteum function after follicle aspiration for oocyte retrieval. Fertil Steril 1981; 36:565–572

[9] Smitz J, Devroey P, Camus M, Deschacht J, Khan I, Staessen C, Van Waesberghe L, Wisanto A, Van Steirteghem AC The luteal phase and early pregnancy after combined GnRH-agonist/HMG treatment for superovulation in IVF or GIFT , Hum Reprod. 1988; 5:585-90.

[10] Elter K, Nelson LR Use of third generation gonadotropin releasing hormone antagonists in in vitro fertilization–embryo transfer: a review. Obstet Gynecol Surv 2001; 56:576–88.

[11] Beckers NGM, Macklon NS, Eijkemans MJC, et al. Comparison of the nonsupplemented luteal phase characteristics after recombinant (r)HCG, rLH or GnRH agonist for oocyte maturation in IVF. Hum Reprod 2002 ; 17: (Suppl. 1):55.

[12] Beckers NG, Macklon NS, Eijkemans MJ, et al. Nonsupplemented luteal phase characteristics after the administration of recombinant human chorionic gonadotropin, recombinant luteinizing hormone, or gonadotropin-releasing hormone (GnRH) agonist to induce final oocyte maturation in in vitro fertilization patients after ovarian

* Corresponding Author

stimulation with recombinant follicle-stimulating hormone and GnRH antagonist cotreatment. J Clin Endocrinol Metab 2003; 88:4186–92.

[13] Penarrubia J, Balasch J, Fabregues F, et al. Human chorionic gonadotrophin luteal support overcomes luteal phase inadequacy after gonadotrophin releasing hormone agonist-induced ovulation in gonadotrophin stimulated cycles. Hum Reprod 1998; 13:3315–18.

[14] Albano C, Grimbizis G, Smitz J, et al. The luteal phase of nonsupplemented cycles after ovarian superovulation with human menopausal gonadotropin and the gonadotropin releasing hormone antagonist Cetrorelix. Fertil Steril 1998: 70:357–9.

[15] Fatemi HM The luteal phase after 3 decades of IVF Reproductive BioMedicine Online, 2009 , : 19, S 4, 1 - 13

[16] Friedler S, Gilboa S, Schachter M, et al. Luteal phase characteristics following GnRH antagonist or agonist treatment – a comparative study. Reprod Biomed Online 2006; 12:27–32

[17] Soliman S, Daya S, Collins J, Hughes EG The role of luteal support in infertility treatments: a meta-analysis of randomized trials. Fertil Steril 1994 ; 61:1068–76

[18] Pritts E, Atwood A Luteal phase support in infertility treat- ment: a meta-analysis of the randomized trials. Hum Reprod1 2002; 7:2287–99

[19] Daya S, Gunby J Luteal phase support in assisted reproduc-tion cycles. Cochrane Database Syst Rev, 2004; CD004830.

[20] Nosarka S, Kruger T, Siebert I, et al. Luteal phase support in in vitro fertilization: metaanalysis of randomized trials. Gynecol Obstet Invest 2005; 60:67–74.

[21] van der Linden M, Buckingham K, Farquhar C, Kremer JAM, Metwally M. Luteal phase support for assisted reproduction cycles. Cochrane Database of Systematic Reviews 2011, Issue 10. Art. No.: CD009154. DOI:

[22] Ottoson UB, Johansson BG, Von Schoultz B Subfractions of high-density lipoprotein cholesterol during estrogen replacement therapy: a comparison between progestogens and natural progesterone. American Journal of Obstetrics and Gynecology 1985;151: 746–750.

[23] Penzias AS. Luteal phase support. Fertil Steril 2002; 77:318–323

[24] Levine H, Watson N. Comparison of the pharmacokinetics of Crinone 8% administered vaginally versus Prometrium administered orally in postmenopausal women. Fertil Steril 2000;73:516–21

[25] Daya S Luteal support: Progestogens for pregnancy protection Maturitas 2009, 65: Supplement 1, Pages S29-S34

[26] R. Dmitrovic, V. Vlaisavljevic, D. Ivankovic Endometrial growth in early pregnancy after IVF/ET J. Assist. Reprod. Genet. 2008; 25:453-9.

[27] Maxson W.S, Hargrove J.T. Bioavailability of oral micronized progesterone Fertil. Steril., 1985;44 : 622 - 626

[28] Margit M. Janát-Amsbury,Kavita M. Gupta, Caroline D. Kablitz, Drug delivery for in vitrofertilization: Rationale, current strategies and challenges Advanced Drug Delivery Reviews 2009;61: 871 - 882

[29] van Broekhoven F., Backstrom T., Verkes R.J. Oral progesterone decreases saccadic eye velocity and increases sedation in women Psychoneuroendocrinology, 2006;31 : 1190 - 1199

[30] Bulletti, D. de Ziegler, C. Flamigni, E. Giacomucci, V. Polli, G. Bolelli et al. Targeted drug delivery in gynaecology: the first uterine pass effect Hum. Reprod., 1997; 12:1073 - 1079

[31] Cicinelli E., De Ziegler D., Bulletti C., M.G. Matteo, Schonauer L.M., Galantino P. Direct transport of progesterone from vagina to uterus Obstet. Gynecol., 2000; 95: 403 - 406

[32] Tavaniotou A., Smitz J., Bourgain C., Devroey P. Comparison between different routes of progesterone administration as luteal phase support in infertility treatments Hum. Reprod. Updat., 2000,6: 139 - 148

[33] Chakravarty BN, Shirazee HH, Dam P, Goswami SK, Chatterjee R, Ghosh S. Oral dydrogesterone versus intravaginal micronised progesterone as luteal phase support in assisted reproductive technology (ART) cycles: results of a randomised study.J Steroid Biochem Mol Biol. 2005 ; 97:416-20.

[34] Patki A, Pawar VC. Modulating fertility outcome in assisted reproductive technologies by the use of dydrogesterone. Gynecol Endocrinol. 2007 Suppl 1:68-72.

[35] Friedler S, Raziel A, Schachter M, Strassburger D, Bukovsky I, Ron-El R. Luteal support with micronized progesterone following in-vitro fertilization using a down-regulation protocol with gonadotrophin-releasing hormone agonist: a comparative study between vaginal and oral administration. Hum Reprod. 1999 ;14:1944-8.

[36] Bacq Y, Sapey T.,. Bréchot M.C, Pierre F.,. Fignon A and. Dubois F, Intrahepatic cholestasis of pregnancy: a French prospective study, Hepatology 26 (1997), pp. 358–364

[37] Licciardi FL, Kwiatkowski A, Noyes NL, et al. Oral versus intramuscular progesterone for in vitro fertilization: a prospective randomized study. Fertil Steril 1999; 71:614–618

[38] Abate A, Perino M, Abate FG, et al. Intramuscular versus vaginal administration of progesterone for luteal phase support after in vitro fertilization and embryo transfer. A comparative randomized study. Clin Exp Obstet Gynecol 1999; 26:203–206

[39] Propst AM, Hill JA, Ginsburg ES, et al. A randomized study comparing crinone 8% and intramuscular progesterone supplementation in in vitro fertilization-embryo transfer cycles. Fertil Steril 2001; 76:1144–1149

[40] Costabile L, Gerli S, Manna C, Rossetti D, Di Renzo GC, Unfer V. A prospective randomized study comparing intramuscular progesterone and 17alpha-hydroxyprogesterone caproate in patients undergoing in vitro fertilization-embryo transfer cycles. Fertil Steril. 2001 Aug;76(2):394-6

[41] Unfer V, Casini ML, Costabile L, Gerli S, Baldini D, Di Renzo GC. 17 alpha-hydroxyprogesterone caproate versus intravaginal progesterone in IVF-embryo transfer cycles: a prospective randomized study. Reprod Biomed Online. 2004;9(1):17-21.

[42] Doody K, Shamma FN, Paulson RJ, et al. Endometrin for luteal phase support in a randomized, controlled, open label, prospective IVF clinical trial using a combination of menopur and bravelle. Fertil Steril 2007; 87(S2):S24

[43] Yanushpoisky E, Hurwitz S, Greenberg L, et al. Comparison of crinone 8% intravaginal gel and intramuscular progesterone supplementation for in vitro fertilization/embryo transfer in women under age 40: interim analysis of a prospective randomized trial. Fertil Steril 2008; 89:458–467.

[44] Levy T., Gurevitch S., Bar-Hava I., Ashkenazi J., Magazanik A.,. Homburg R et al. Pharmacokinetics of natural progesterone administered in the form of a vaginal tablet Hum. Reprod., 1999, 14: 606 - 610

[45] Germond M, Capelli P., Bruno G, Vesnaver S, Senn A., Rouge N ,. Biollaz J, Comparison of the efficacy and safety of two formulations of micronized progesterone (Ellios™and Utrogestan™) used as luteal phase support after in vitro fertilization Fertil Steril 77: 313-315 ,2002

[46] Yu Ng EH , Chan CCW, Tang OS, Ho PC A randomized comparison of side effects and patient convenience between Cyclogest suppositories and Endometrin tablets used for luteal phase support in IVF treatment European Journal of Obstetrics & Gynecology and Reproductive Biology 2007; 131: 182–188

[47] Ludwig M, Schwartz P, Babahan B, Katalinic A, Weiss JM, Felberbaum R, Al-Hasani S, Diedrich K. Luteal phase support using either Crinone 8% or Utrogest: results of a prospective, randomized study. Eur J Obstet Gynecol Reprod Biol. 2002 103:48-52.

[48] Kleinstein J. Efficacy and tolerability of vaginal progesterone capsules (Utrogest™ 200) compared with progesterone gel (Crinone™ 8%) for luteal phase support during assisted reproduction. Fertil Steril 2005;83:1641–9.

[49] Silverberg KM, Vaughn TC, Hansard LJ, Burger NZ, Minter T.Vaginal (Crinone 8%) gel vs. intramuscular progesterone in oil for luteal phase support in in vitro fertilization: a large prospective trial. Fertil Steril. 2012;97:344-8.

[50] Polyzos NP, Messini CI, Papanikolaou EG, Mauri D, Tzioras S, Badawy A, Messinis IE. Vaginal progesterone gel for luteal phase support in IVF/ICSI cycles: a meta-analysis. Fertil Steril. 2010 94:2083-7.

[51] Pirard C, Donnez J, Loumaye E. GnRH agonist as luteal phase support in assisted reproduction technique cycles: results of a pilot study. Hum Reprod 2006; 21:1894–1900

[52] Tesarik J, Hazout A, Mendoza-Tesarik R, et al. Beneficial effect of luteal-phase GnRH agonist administration on embryo implantation after ICSI in both GnRH agonist- and antagonist-treated ovarian stimulation cycles. Hum Reprod 2006; 21:2572–2579

[53] Ata B, Yakin K, Balaban B, et al. GnRH agonist protocol administration in the luteal phase in ICSI-ET cycles stimulated with the long GnRH agonist protocol: a randomized, controlled double blind study. Hum Reprod 2008; 23:668–673

[54] Tesarik J, Hazout A, Mendoza C Enhancement of embryo developmental potential by a single administration of GnRH agonist at the time of implantation. Hum Reprod 2004 19:1176–80

[55] Pirard C, Donnez J, Loumaye E GnRH agonist as novel luteal support: results of a randomised, parallel group, feasibility study using intranasal administration of buserelin. Hum Reprod 2005 20:1798–804.

[56] Hughes JN, Cedrin-Durnerin I, Bstandig B, et al. Administration of gonadotropin-releasing hormone agonist during the luteal phase of the GnRH-antagonist IVF cycles. Hum Reprod 2006; 21 (Suppl. 1):O-007.

[57] Kyrou D, Kolibianakis EM, Fatemi HM, Tarlatzi TB, Devroey P, Tarlatzis BC. Increased live birth rates with GnRH agonist addition for luteal support in ICSI/IVF cycles: a systematic review and meta-analysis. Hum Reprod Update. 2011 ;17:734-40.

[58] Mochtar MH, Hogerzeil HV, Mol BW Progesterone alone versus progesterone combined with HCG as luteal support in GnRHa/HMG induced IVF cycles: a randomized clinical trial.Hum Reprod 1996; 11:1602–5

[59] Fujimoto A, Osuga Y, Fujiwara T, et al. Human chorionic gonadotrophin combined with progesterone for luteal support improves pregnancy rate in patients with low late-midluteal es-tradiol levels in IVF cycles. J Assist Reprod Genet 2002 19:550–4.

[60] Ludwig M, Finas A, Katalinic A, et al. (2001) Prospective, random-ized study to evaluate the success rates using hCG, vaginal pro-gesterone or a combination of both for luteal phase support. Acta Obstet Gynecol Scand 80:574–82

[61] Smitz J, Devroey P, Braeckmans P, Camus M, Khan L, Staessen C, et al. Management of failed cycles in an IVF/GIFT programme with the combination of a GnRH analogue and hMG. Hum Reprod 1987;2:309–14.

[62] Fatemi HM, Popovic-Todorovic B, Papanikolaou E, Donoso P,Devroey P. An update of luteal phase support in stimulated IVF cycles.Hum Reprod Update 2007;13:581.

[63] Ghanem M E., Ehab E. Sadek, Elboghdady L. A.. Helal A S, Gamal Anas, Eldiasty A Bakre N I., Houssen M .The effect of luteal phase support protocol on cycle outcome and luteal phase hormone profile in long agonist protocol intracytoplasmic sperm injection cycles: a randomized clinical trial , Fertility and Sterility 2009 92: 486-493

[64] Var T, Tonguc EA, Doğanay M, Gulerman C, Gungor T, Mollamahmutoglu L. A comparison of the effects of three different luteal phase support protocols on in vitro fertilization outcomes: a randomized clinical trial. Fertil Steril. 2011 95:985-9.

[65] Gelbaya TA, KyrgiouM, Tsoumpou I, Nardo LG. The use of estradiol for luteal phase support in in vitro fertilization/intracytoplasmic sperminjec- tion cycles: a systematic review and meta-analysis. Fertil Steril 2008;90: 2116-25.

[66] Jee BC, Suh CS, Kim SH, Kim YB, Moon SY. Effects of estradiol supplementation during the luteal phase of in vitro fertilization cycles: a meta-analysis Fertil Steril. 2010 93:428-36

[67] Williams SG, Oehninger S, Gibbons WE, et al. Delaying the initiation of progesterone supplementation results in decreased pregnancy rates after in vitro fertilization: a randomized prospective study. Fertil Steril 2001; 76:1140–3.

[68] Mochtar MH, Van Wely M, Van der Veen F. Timing luteal phase support in GnRH agonist down-regulated IVF/embryo transfer cycles. Hum Reprod 2006; 21:905–908

[69] Schmidt KL, Ziebe S, Popovic B, et al. Progesterone supplementation during early gestation after in vitro fertilization has no effect on the delivery rate. Fertil Steril 2001; 75:337–341

[70] Aboulghar MA, Amin Y, Al-Inany H, et al. Prospective randomized study comparing luteal phase support for ICSI patients up to the first ultrasound compared with an additional three weeks. Hum Reprod 2008; 33:857–862

[71] Andersen AN, Popovic-Todorovic B, Schmidt KT, et al. Progesterone supplementation during early gestations after IVF or ICSI has no effect on the delivery rates: a randomized controlled trial. Hum Reprod 2002; 17:357–361